More Praise for *Welcoming Consciousness*

"Once in a great while a concept comes along that seems so radical that it is at the same time both revolutionary and impossible, yet profoundly true. Such a concept that turns current thinking upside down and opens a window on our understanding of human development is presented in *Welcoming Consciousness*. Dr. McCarty has synthesized decades of prenatal and perinatal psychology's clinical findings and her own observations of babies and children to bring us a new way of thinking about what it means to be fully human. A must read for anyone who cares about infants and children and the development of their full potential, this book is a recipe for helping us plumb our depths at any age."

— MARTI GLENN, PH.D., founding president, Santa Barbara Graduate Institute, Graduate Studies in Prenatal and Perinatal Psychology

"*Welcoming Consciousness* is an exceptional asset to the growing understanding of both the exquisite awareness and delicate vulnerabilities that babies bring with them into the world. All those interested in enhancing the well-being of pre-nates, newborns, and toddlers will benefit from the wisdom that Dr. McCarty shares from her vast clinical experience and research."

— PETER A LEVINE, PH.D., co-author, *Trauma Through a Child's Eyes, Awakening the Ordinary Miracle of Healing*

"I highly recommend *Welcoming Consciousness*, its perspective on integrating mind, body and spirit truly has the potential to change the world. We have all been indoctrinated with the belief that the character of our lives is preprogrammed in the genes. However, a radically new understanding in science now reveals that it is our perceptions of the world that controls genes and programs our behavior. In *Welcoming Consciousness*, Wendy Anne McCarty, PhD, offers important insights into how pre- and perinatal experiences provide for the most influential perceptions that shape one's life. Dr. McCarty's synthesis of leading edge biomedical science, current psychology and the awareness acquired through her professional practice provides an important contribution to our understanding of the human experience. I thoroughly enjoyed this book."

— BRUCE H. LIPTON, PH.D., cell biologist, author, *The Biology of Belief: Unleashing the Power of Consciousness, Matter and Miracles*

"Wendy Anne McCarty is the emerging voice in the field of pre and perinatal psychology. Her work with babies is that of grace unfolding. All therapists would do well to become familiar with how she works with little ones."

— MICHAEL SHEA, PH.D., biodynamic craniosacral therapist, international trainer, author, *Biodynamic Craniosacral Therapy*

"Wendy Anne McCarty has taken a bold and important step forward in *Welcoming Consciousness* by integrating both theory and practical approaches to strengthening babies' innate connection with the intuitive intelligence of their spirit. The processes discussed provides approaches that can enhance children's intuitive awareness and build a new foundation for continuing growth including a deeper sense of care and connection to all living things."

— ROLLIN MCCRATY, PH.D., director of research, Institute of HeartMath

"In her groundbreaking book *Welcoming Consciousness*, Dr. McCarty convincingly brings prenatal and perinatal psychology into the 21st century. In weaving together astonishing clinical stories, quantum physics, holographic theory, psychology, and philosophy, she introduces an integrative early development model that portrays babies as conscious, aware, and sentient beings from the beginning of life. This book is a MUST for anyone involved in pregnancy, birth, and supporting babies and young children."

— PAUL BRENNER, MD, PH.D., obstetrician and psychotherapist, author, *Buddha in the Waiting Room*

"This unique work of Wendy Anne McCarty is an intellectual milestone--the first attempt to integrate theory and practice of pre- and perinatal psychology with other early developmental theories. Adept in positive appreciation of the currently separate fields and gifted in discerning both shortcomings and greater potentials, Wendy also understands the imperative to move beyond a fixed Newtonian view of reality to a comprehensive science of human consciousness. Considering these many talents, I cannot think of a better person to handle a sensitive project of this scope. Or one who could wrap it up in just 129 pages followed by 34 pages of topical bibliographies to satisfy any scholar's yearning for more…"

— DAVID CHAMBERLAIN, PH.D., past president of APPPAH, author, *The Mind of Your Newborn Baby*

"*Welcoming Consciousness* explores the sentient nature of life itself and more to the point of each new, emerging human being. We are both mind and matter, wave and partial, spirit and form, Wendy provides us a bridge, a way of looking and integrating our conscious, formless, quantum self and our biological, material, physical self. *Welcoming Consciousness* is clear, provocative and deeply human."

— MICHAEL MENDIZZA, founder, Touch the Future, www.ttfuture.org, co-author with Joseph Chilton Pearce, *Magical Parent-Magical Child*

"What a wonderful book Dr. McCarty has written. From the moment I picked it up, I could not put it down. Dr. McCarty succeeds in introducing an integrative model of early human experience that takes our understanding of early human development, pre and perinatal psychology, and healing to higher and more potent levels. Her book tells of her evolving journey through traditional ways of viewing babies into pre and perinatal psychology and experiential spirituality. She incorporates theories and clinical cases from a wide variety of practitioners, writers, and healers, weaving theory and practice with balance and grace. In her model, Dr. McCarty reintegrates our basic, sentient nature into our developmental theories and clinical practices. She posits a dual source of awareness, one associated with the biological human self and another with the transcendent self, having awareness preceding conception and surviving death. This is a marvelous book. A unique contribution and a must read! It will transform your practice and your understanding of life."

— WILLIAM R. EMERSON, PH.D., co-president, Association of Prenatal and Perinatal Psychology and Health, pioneer in prenatal and perinatal psychology, director of Emerson Training Seminars

"Dr. Wendy Anne McCarty has given us an amazing work by giving words to experiences that have origins from preverbal time or that time before any of us had words. She welcomes consciousness by giving respect to early experience that so many of us know in our heart of hearts to be true. For those who are on the edge of discovering consciousness prior to the development of our nervous systems, she helps us stretch our thinking in ways that opens the doors into this new paradigm. Thank you, Wendy. "

— RAYMOND CASTELLINO, D.C., clinic director, BEBA, director, Castellino Prenatal and Birth Training

"I am thrilled that this book has been written. Wendy Anne McCarty's material is essential for understanding our prenatal beginnings and how they continually replicate in our life and relationships. I highly recommend it to everyone interested in their own self-help process and to all those who work in the healthcare field. It is on the list for every Resonance Repatterning practitioner to read."

—CHLOE FAITH WORDSWORTH, founder, Resonance Repatterning(TM) System

"What a tour de force! I enjoyed *Welcoming Consciousness* immensely and found it most impressive. It's great the way you have set the evidence of experience into a philosophical background. As a fellow researcher and writer in the field, my favorite parts were the stories and examples and your own experiences. Yet, the theoretical underpinnings you provide help substantiates the reality of the incoming soul."

— ELISABETH HALLETT, author, *Soul Trek; Stories of the Unborn Soul: The Mystery and Delight of Pre-Birth Communication*

"As a healthcare practitioner for 25 years specializing in CranioSacral Therapy the question of how to communicate our conscious and sentient wholeness to other healthcare providers or the public who do not have that orientation has placed me in the category of '... one of those wacky metaphysical types.' Those human beings, who have experienced that part of their nature, know empirically of its validity and those have not, will often dismiss it. My work has guided me to place implicit trust in a fetus and newborn's capacity to understand complex emotions and situations. When working with these families, witnessing a parent's newfound cognition of their baby's comprehension is remarkable. In the field of Prenatal and Perinatal Psychology, there seems to be a gap between the subjective experiences and academic writing and research regarding consciousness. Dr. McCarty's new book, *Welcoming Consciousness: Supporting Babies' Wholeness From the Beginning of Life* is the first working theoretical model to attempt to bridge the chasm between the two paradigms. Dr. McCarty begins to bring a holistic model of infant development that is inclusive of consciousness with rationales that are based from the diverse and dynamic fields of physics, psychology, and spirituality. It inspires me to pursue the topic more vigorously and gives me great hope for healing the wound in our culture perpetuated by separation of consciousness from the mind and body."

— JENNIFER ABSEY, R.N., C.M.T.

Welcoming
Consciousness

Welcoming Consciousness

Supporting Babies' Wholeness
From the Beginning of Life

Wendy Anne McCarty, PhD

An Integrated Model of Early Development

Wondrous Beginnings Publishing
315 Meigs Road, #A306, Santa Barbara, CA 93109
www.wondrousbeginnings.com

The author is grateful for permission to use the following previously copyrighted material: The Resonant Heart" by Rollin McCraty, PhD, Raymond Trevor Bradley & Dana Tomasino, published in Shift: At the Frontiers of Consciousness No. 5 (Dec. 2004-Feb. 2005), is reprinted by permission of the authors (www.heartmath.org) and the Institute of Noetic Sciences (www.noetic. org). Copyright 2005, all rights reserved.

Cover design, book design and Dr. McCarty's photo by Lynda Rae, www.auroradesignstudio.com

McCarty, Wendy Anne.
    Welcoming consciousness : supporting babies'
    wholeness from the beginning of life : an integrated
    model of early development / Wendy Anne McCarty.
      p. cm.
    Includes bibliographical references
    Originally published: ISBN 0-9760658-5-1

    1. Developmental psychology. 2. Consciousness.
    3. Fetal behavior. I. Title.

BF713.M336 2006   155.2

First ePrinting, PDF, 2004
Revised ePrinting, PDF, 2005
Revised and expanded Print edition, 2009
    ISBN 978-0-9760658-6-9

Acknowledgments

I am deeply grateful to the New Earth Foundation for their vision and for their valuing the importance of re-constellating our early development models to include consciousness and our sentient spiritual nature. Without their support, this book and the research behind it would not have been possible. Special thanks to Lorna McLeod, director of NEF, who guided me through this project.

I am very grateful to Carolyn Kenny, founding academic director, Santa Barbara Graduate Institute, who mentored me in newer and more integrative expressions of research and writing during this project and who served as my project advisor. Thank you. I also want to thank Shannon Venable for her editorial contribution and Lynda Rae for her additional editorial support, beautiful book cover and book design.

I am deeply grateful to Marti Glenn and Ken Bruer for inviting me to help create and birth Santa Barbara Graduate Institute and to co-found the Prenatal and Perinatal Psychology Program with Marti. This opportunity has challenged me to explore more deeply the integration of early development models and prenatal and perinatal psychology and now ten years later has evolved into the new disciple of primary psychology and our 12 guiding principles. What an adventure, Marti!

I want to acknowledge and thank Ray Castellino, with whom I co-founded BEBA, the non-profit clinic providing PPN-oriented therapeutic work with babies and their families in 1993. During our five years as co-therapists, I learned a great deal from Ray. It was a special time of collaboration and development of the work.

Other mentors, teachers, pioneers, and colleagues I want to give a special thanks and recognition to are William Emerson, Franklyn Sills, Peter Levine, Chloe Wordsworth, David Chamberlain, Thomas Verny, Jenny Wade, Rollin McCraty, Michael Shea, Joseph Chilton Pearce, and Walter Makichen. I am grateful to all those pioneers who founded and have participated in the development of prenatal and perinatal psychology and The Association of Prenatal and Perinatal Psychology and

Health. Special acknowledgement to B. J. Lyman, the current editor of our field's journal, JOPPPH, and the former chair of the Prenatal and Perinatal Psychology Program at SBGI for six years.

On a personal note, I'm deeply grateful to my friends and family, especially Ginny, Patsy, Harvey, Jennifer, Leslie, Annie, Sharon, Daniel, Paul, Thomas, Terry, and Bill who held the space for the project and for me from pre-conception to birthing of this material. Your support has meant so much to me. I am profoundly grateful to Lazaris for reaching out a hand and lighting my way home—a wondrous beginning.

I am deeply grateful and feel blessed to have the privilege of working with all the families, babies, children, and adults who have taught me so much about who we are, our dignity, our character, and our deepest drive to love, heal and connect with our truth. Thank you so much for allowing me to share your stories so that others can be touched and awaken more of themselves.

My deepest gratitude goes to my parents. I know they loved, wanted, and valued me from the beginning. Precious gifts. I want to acknowledge how wonderful my mom was during all the years of my PPN training and my exploration of my PPN experiences. Time and time again, she patiently and lovingly allowed me to ask her questions, let me tell her my stories of re-connection with these experiences, and just loved me through it all. Looking back, one of the most healing elements in my journey was Mom's ability to share what she remembered and how she had felt and to say, "I'm sorry…I wish it was different…I didn't know…." She taught me so much by her ability to allow and hold my story without falling off the edge into guilt or shame, or needing to push my truths away if they were painful ones. So much of the early wounding was in feeling separation in my experience, and, in her quiet way, she helped me feel the connection I had missed and brought us closer together. It was wonderful. Love you always, Mom. Thank you with all my heart.

Contents

Shh…
Let your hearts be still
Come quietly
Come softly
Come soon
Come
To a new world

— Bill

Chapter I

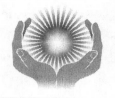

Introduction

"They don't think I'm a person. I *know* I am."

This experience and statement captures a core theme echoed throughout decades of clinical reports from the field of prenatal and perinatal psychology. This particular report comes from Emily under hypnosis as she described her experience in the newborn nursery to Dr. David Chamberlain (1999b, p. 80). Dr. Chamberlain has been gathering stories and research concerning the sentient nature of babies in the womb and at birth for over thirty years. His body of work as a practicing prenatal and perinatal psychologist and researcher, including two books and over fifty published articles, is an integral contribution to the emerging field of prenatal and perinatal psychology (PPN). In his article "The Significance of Birth Memories," he voices what has been reported repeatedly in the PPN literature, namely that "all birth memories are imbued with a sense of identity" (p.79).

I believe the most important step in creating an integrated model of early development is to reconstitute our sentient spiritual nature as our fundamental nature, with our human self as an aspect or expression of our sentient self. When we recognize, acknowledge, and support the sentient being entering human form, we reconstellate our theories, assessments, interventions, parenting practices, and foundational ways of being with babies to support wholeness from the beginning of life.

Most people, not having been exposed to the PPN literature or lacking their own reconnection with their life in the womb or at birth, might find these statements disorienting and unbelievable. For those of us in the early development community trained in mainstream infant development theory and research, the notion of a newborn being capable of having a sense of self-identity is contrary to contemporary conceptualizations of young infants.

One fundamental tenet of traditional early development theory has been that the human infant's experience is merged (fused) with that of the mother and the physical environment. This perspective rests on the prevalent view of the human being as a biologically based entity and as viewed behaviorally. Babies in the womb, at birth, and during the early weeks and months of life are seen as incapable of reflection, sense of self, meaningful understanding of language, or of conscious communication. Within this perspective, a primary developmental task of infants during the first two years of life is to develop a sense of self, separate from their environment and separate from mother. Within this model, consciousness and a conscious sense of self is perceived to emerge out of the developing human brain over a period of months and years.

A very different view of early development and capabilities

has been emerging over the last three decades as clinical findings from the field of prenatal and perinatal psychology have mapped out the experience of our earliest development from *the baby's point of view*. This vantage point gives rise to a very different perspective and view of SELF during life in the womb and early infancy. Prenatal and perinatal psychology findings suggest we are conscious sentient beings from the beginning of life and that we exist as sentient beings prior to physical life and are functioning as such from the beginning of human existence.

Thus, the traditional infant development literature and the prenatal and perinatal psychology clinical findings appear to have very different orientations, perspectives, and descriptions of infants. Each of these traditions also has its own various ensuing implications concerning how best to care for the infant and support optimal infant development, which can appear significantly different from one another. At the core of the differences appears the question of our basic nature.

This dissonance and these paradoxes have fueled my explorations as clinician, educator, and researcher for the past fifteen years. This book represents my attempt to address and to resolve core paradoxes and apparent disagreements between mainstream infant development models and the growing evidence from prenatal and perinatal psychology by bringing them together in a model that can hold the essence of the full spectrum of perspectives. In this process, I hope to create a more accurate and coherent narrative of early development that begins with the conception of a new human being.

My decades of exploration is a tapestry woven of threads from my own personal experiences, professional education, and clinical experience, as well as my work and dialogue with members of the early development and prenatal and perinatal psychology communities. Thus my conclusions represent a synergy of these various perspectives. The book is intended for a wide audience, from those new to prenatal and perinatal psychology literature to seasoned early development theorists and especially to everyone working with young families.

Many of the ideas have a foundation in previous work by others, yet some of the ways I thread ideas together could be considered quite speculative at this point. This model benefits from the spectrum of theoretical thought and is grounded in my direct clinical experience with adults, children, and babies.

My purpose here, stated more specifically, is to introduce an integrative model of early human experience, learning, development, and caretaking (pre-conception through early infancy) that includes our sentient nature by focusing on bridging and integrating several fields such as current infant development theories, new clinical research with babies that incorporates consciousness, prenatal and perinatal psychology, parenting practices, and several notions within the new physics sciences. This book is meant as the beginning of this process.

I sketch aspects of the new model and provide an exploratory articulation that can feed new thought, new research, and professional investigation in early development theory and application. Key concepts are presented and clinical examples provided; yet the intent is not meant as an in-depth treatment or a review of the literature of any one aspect.

When presenting an area or finding, I cite one or two authors who are examples or representative of the material, rather than the larger list of references in that arena. I include an extensive bibliography for further exploration in the Appendix Bibliography. The discussion relating these intricate theoretical issues to everyday, practical applications of how we conceive, carry, birth, and raise babies and young children is introduced. In further articulations, I plan to address specific aspects of and issues raised by the model in more depth, as well as further descriptions and implications of the PPN-oriented clinical work with babies and young children.

Chapter II

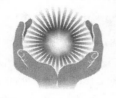

Evolving Beliefs, Conceptions, and Perceptions

As I look back over the last twenty-five years of my clinical practice, core themes emerge that seem pertinent to our discussion here. One theme is the power that my beliefs have on what I (a) conceive to be possible or true and (b) perceive when I am observing and interacting with a baby. I see how my beliefs profoundly shape me as a practitioner working with babies and as a researcher.

In 2003, I viewed a Discovery Health television program, *The Placebo Effect*. In one segment, Dr. Albert Mason relates his story of decades ago when as a young doctor he saw a patient with what he believed were thousands of warts on his body. He had been trained in hypnosis and knew that warts were curable with the use of hypnosis. He proceeded to hypnotize the patient and the warts successfully healed. When his attending physician later saw the patient, he told Dr. Mason that those had not been warts on the patient, but rather a manifestation of a genetic, incurable disease. The success of the case had been reported in a national magazine and many suffering from this debilitating disease came for the young doctor's hypnosis treatment.

Dr. Mason relates that although he treated many others with the same ailment utilizing similar hypnotic suggestions, none ever had any beneficial effect. Looking back over this experience years later, Dr. Mason suggests the reason the hypnotic treatments never worked effectively again is that *he no longer believed it was possible.* He felt he was only play-acting the treatment. By the way, the documentary crew located his original patient who related his condition had remained healed for the thirty years since treatment.

This story moves me deeply and speaks to themes in my own exploration. What are my beliefs about early human development? What is possible? How has my culture, family, education, and training shaped me as a practitioner in terms of what I conceive and even perceive when I am with a baby? What is healing and therapeutic in this new context? What do I believe to be true in the face of my direct experience and what I have been taught to be true? How do we know something is true? In the following section, I share pieces of my own journey moving from a traditional Western view of birth and babies into the world of prenatal and perinatal psychology and returning to integrate them. The discussion also acts as a brief introduction to the PPN field.

My Journey

When I graduated from college in 1973, I worked as a nurse at the University of Kentucky Medical Center's "labor and delivery unit." I learned and participated in high-tech, high-intervention Western birth methods at this teaching hospital. I thought that was "the way to deliver babies." In my next job, I headed up a team of nurses and social workers in a high-risk maternity home visitation program. In 1976, I participated in a new research NCAST project through a live-satellite learning program focusing on the new mother-infant assessments during feeding time and teaching sequences and infant states. It was a very exciting time in infant research and in intervention programs, with new research on parent-infant reciprocity and attunement and infant stimulation programs blossoming.

In 1977, I returned to school and received a master's degree in Child Development and Family Studies, focusing on infant development. For my master's thesis, I carried out a longitudinal study of couples having their first babies and examined certain aspects of the transition to parenthood (Wong, 1979). I was most drawn to the counseling side of working with families and went on to get my doctorate from the University of Southern California in Counseling Psychology. My research again focused on the transition to parenthood (McCarty-Wong, 1986). My counseling orientation was primarily humanistic-existential, with five years of training in Gestalt therapy. I opened my private marriage and family therapy practice in 1986.

At the same time, in my personal life the "transition to parenthood" was not happening for me and for my husband. Upon discovering that my husband was infertile, we began a seven-year journey immersed in the infertility maze, with sperm donors, artificial inseminations, surgeries, in-vitro fertilization, and a failed adoption. I have a great deal of compassion for those finding themselves in that journey. These experiences gave me an inside view of high-tech conception which is such a vital topic when we bring it into an integrated model's understanding. During those years, I took a hiatus from working with families having babies and my psychotherapy practice focused on working with adults.

Prenatal and Perinatal Psychology

In 1988, I received a flier for a conference held by the Prenatal and Perinatal Psychology Association of North America, which later became the Association of Prenatal and Perinatal Psychology and Health (APPPAH). It was intriguing, but very "70's-ish" sounding to me with topics such as the cellular consciousness of the sperm and the egg. I had never heard of prenatal and perinatal psychology before that time, my obstetrical work with birth and my therapy practice up until then were totally separate. Now there was a field that brought both together. It sounded intriguing.

I attended the conference and my rather neatly packaged understanding of the world and babies was graciously turned upside down! During the conference, Dr. William Emerson presented his groundbreaking psychotherapy work with infants that focused on healing birth trauma. I could not even imagine what that meant before I attended the session. What is birth trauma? Psychotherapy with a three-month-old? Dr. Emerson showed a video of a treatment session he had with a young baby. The baby was portraying movement patterns and emotional expressions associated with a difficult portion of his birth. It appeared that he and the baby were having a very intimate mutual communication about it. In that moment, I experienced the baby's depth of presence, his capacity to communicate with and understand Dr. Emerson's communication with him. Dr. Emerson quietly acknowledged to the baby how similar the baby's present experience felt to a particularly difficult time in his birth, empathizing with the baby's experience. At one point the baby was in a deep and quiet stillness as he looked into Dr. Emerson's eyes and I was filled with the sense that the baby's expression was one of gratitude. His expression appeared to be conveying his appreciation of Dr. Emerson's "being with him in this place," and communicating in this way with him. I saw something in this interchange and in the baby's expression that I had never seen in babies before and *it changed me.*

I believe I was open to seeing this because I was in the *presence of someone who held it to be possible.* Dr. Emerson not only held it as possible, but also had been unraveling for over twenty years the meaning of what babies have been expressing for so long about their prenatal and birth experiences and sentient nature. He had been treating adults with PPN-related issues for years and was inspired to work with children's PPN-oriented issues. His work subsequently progressed to working with infants to resolve their early trauma (Emerson, 1998, 1999a, 1999b, 2001a, 2001a).

The 1988 conference was a watershed of new ideas and new experiences. Some of them were exciting, some seemingly far-fetched, and some just disorienting. During the conference, I learned that the field's roots were grounded in therapeutic work with adults. Therapists had unexpectedly witnessed clients discover the origins of their psychological and physical issues in their prenatal and birth experiences. In an effort to understand this uncharted territory, they began to meet and the field grew from there. By the late 1980's, it had expanded into a multidisciplinary field "dedicated to the in-depth exploration of the psychological dimension of human reproduction and pregnancy and the mental and emotional development of the unborn and newborn child" (*The Journal of Prenatal and Perinatal Psychology and Health*'s purpose statement).

- The field focused on the prenatal and birth process and experience directly, as well as on the understanding and treatment of children, adolescents, and adults exhibiting constrictive-to-traumatic patterns rooted in their PPN experience. Basic concepts included:
- How we are conceived, carried, birthed, and greeted matters greatly.
- We are conscious, sentient beings communicating meaningfully from the beginning of life.
- What happens to us during conception, life in the womb, and at birth is remembered and sets in motion life patterns that affect us over the life span.
- A wide variety of therapeutic endeavors and findings with adults, children, and babies collectively converge revealing patterns of effects from a variety of events and medical interventions during the prenatal and perinatal period.

I was reeling from this conference. None of this fit with my previous understanding of pregnancy, birth, babies, or my own understanding of me! What was real? What was true? Why had I not previously seen what I saw in that baby in that moment with William?

Recently, I was in a class and had an experience that brings this point home. Dr. Rollin McCraty, the Director of Research at the Institute of HeartMath and lead researcher in the extensive research on heart intelligence, gave a class at Santa Barbara Graduate Institute that I attended. He introduced an exercise in which we were to watch a video of a basketball game with two teams, one with white shirts, and the other with black shirts. The goal was to successfully count the number of times the white shirt team members bounce passed the basketball to each other. Afterwards he asked us how many bounce passes did we see? In the class of 15-20 people, we gave responses from zero to seven! I was relieved when he said four was the correct number, for I had counted four and I valued my honed observational skills!

Then he asked, "Did anyone see anything else?" One person in the room was confident that she had seen something else. Another person thought perhaps she had seen something. He asked her what she had seen? She said, "I saw a gorilla walk across the basketball court." One person out of the entire group saw the gorilla walk across the court! After this revelation, we watched the video and at that point, we all saw the gorilla. It was an effective exercise to demonstrate the notion of selective perception. Rollin had effectively oriented our attention to the basketball players and that is what we consciously focused on, allowing the other significant gorilla image be unattended to and therefore unrealized. Yet, as soon as the gorilla's presence was brought to our attention consciously, we perceived it.

This simple exercise illustrates an important point in looking at our understanding of babies and early development. How we are taught to see babies, our morphogenetic fields and our culture, how we are treated as babies—all of these contribute to where we place our attention, to select what we make real and what meaning we give to those perceptions. I felt like I had spent my life, my education and professional career observing the basketball game and now William Emerson and others in PPN were asking, "Did you see the gorilla walking across the court?" I turned my attention to learn all I could about the gorilla.

My Prenatal and Perinatal Experiences Revisited

A year later, I began training with Dr. Emerson. During each training module, we did a piece of our own early work. My first birth regression taught me that the family stories of our birth don't always match up with our own experience of birth. We had divided up into pairs to facilitate each other's work. I told my partner that mine was going to be "quick and easy" and that we'd probably be able to break for lunch early. After all, that had been the story of my birth told to me by my mother. "You were two weeks early and even though I thought I wasn't very far along, when I went to the hospital, they informed me I was ready for the delivery room. Shortly thereafter you were born—quick and easy."

During the regression, as I began to go inward, I was stunned by my almost immediate visceral experience of pure terror. I found myself feeling asphyxiated and compressed. I was in an absolute panic to get out. I worked with all my might to move through and I quickly emerged. I experienced visceral memories and sensed a cold, rough hand yanking on my neck and shoulders. I felt very disoriented and groggy. Then I experienced the most existential howl of despair I could imagine. I couldn't get to my mother. They had taken me away. I kept feeling, "what a waste." I felt I had so much love to give her and she wasn't there for me to show her. My heart ached in the timeless period away from her. I remembered feeling so utterly alone and unseen. No one saw ME. It was devastating. After the experience, I kept saying over and over to myself, "I had no idea."

All those years I was a nurse and I had been the one who had participated in these practices, such as immediately taking the baby to the central nursery for "processing." I never got what it was like from the baby's point of view. I never expected to experience what I re-connected with within myself. During the next five years, I experienced forty to fifty sessions of my pre-conception through infancy experiences through a variety of methods and settings: primal regression, guided imagery, hypnosis, craniosacral session, meditation, sand tray work, movement and art therapy, and through spontaneous activations during training and sessions with my clients.

Underlying all of my experiences, I found I had a clear sense of myself. Often I was in the midst of a viscerally intense experience, yet I also had a *witness self* that was experiencing it from a much broader perspective. Depending on the type of orientation or method of work, sometimes I tended to have more somatic, visceral, and even cellular experiences, other times my awareness came from my expanded consciousness perspective. During my own work, I never experienced an interruption of my sense of self and I had an intense yearning for my parents and others to see ME and include ME. I experienced my sentient nature repeatedly. I understood from the inside out what so many others had reported in the PPN literature.

After many of my personal sessions, I would call my mom and ask her to recollect specific aspects of my birth and infancy. I found my experiences repeatedly validated by additional pieces of information she would remember. For example, in one session, I was in a sequence of extension movements, seemingly during my birth when my head was crowning. I was proactively working to be born and then felt myself lose my body energy and float into an unpleasant, groggy, disconnected fog. From that point on, things seemed more to happen to me rather than under my own volition and as I was birthed, I felt disoriented and ineffectual. Afterwards, I called my mom and she remembered they had given her "a whiff of ether at the end there." So there was an external validation of a felt sense of the ether entering my system just before birth.

In these experiences I came to trust the realness, the intensity, and the depth of impact my prenatal and birth experiences had and were continuing to have in my life. I could see the correlating life patterns with *every aspect* of my adult life. It was compelling and it was incredibly healing to do the work. My direct experience during my own work was an integral part of building my new beliefs about prenates and babies and my ability to conceive, perceive, and empathize with the PPN patterns portrayed by people I worked with.

What Children Taught Me

I began seeing young toddlers and children in my practice in 1989, utilizing the prenatal and perinatal psychology framework and what I was learning with Dr. Emerson. I set my office up with over 300-400 sand tray objects—everything that could be a symbol of eggs, sperm, tubes, embryos, fetuses, wombs, cords, placenta, in-out games, hospital scenes, babies, family life, and everyday symbols. I had props to make tunnels and caves, large and small. I developed a mindset that everything they showed me had meaning and my role was to hold their stories sacred and to be with the mystery of it as it unfolded until I understood what their stories were about.

I allowed myself to suspend my earlier training and beliefs about babies and young children and to be open to more of my direct experience of what they were showing me. *Almost every previous belief I had was challenged by what these young children were showing me.* When I began to write later about this work, I titled the publications *What Babies Are Teaching Us,* for they were the ones teaching me.

For the sake of brevity in this book, I will share only a few of these examples to give you a sense of their PPN-oriented memories and how they were still being influenced by their early experiences. I have changed some names for privacy.

Evan's mother asks her six year old, "Do you remember your birth?" He replies, "Sure." She tries to hide her surprise, and asks, "What do you remember?" Evan puts his hands up on the sides of his head and says, "It was really dark and smooshy. It really hurt my head. Then I came out and they handed me to dad. Then dad came to you... did you love me?" She felt a dread. She had felt very guilty that when he was born and brought to her, she was still in so much pain as the episiotomy was repaired that she could not even look at her newborn and had told her husband to take him. She had never told anyone about this because she judged herself harshly for that moment. She then told her son the truth about that moment and said that later when they brought him to her, she fell in love with him. She told him how sorry she was if he felt she had not loved him in that first moment. He said, "Okay" and changed the subject.

Beau was a thirteen-month-old adopted boy who showed no preference for his parents. When he was under distress, he would stop himself from coming to them and distract himself with objects. Within a short time after entering my office, Beau had picked up an object from my open shelves of 300 or more objects and dropped one to the floor. It was a plastic figurine of an actress. I had two figurines of this actress, one in a yellow evening gown and one in a black gown. He chose the one wearing the black gown. The next object was a parent bunny pushing a baby bunny in a carriage. What did these mean?

The parents shared that the adoption had been an open adoption with the birth parents living close by the last month of pregnancy. The four parents decided to all four decorate the baby's room together and the birth couple spent time with their newborn during his first two weeks of life. At two weeks the birth parents signed the paperwork and left on the plane to return home. I asked the mother if Beau had seen photos of his birth mom. She said no, that she was saving them until he was older. I asked if she would bring them to the next session.

Two weeks later, I found out what the actress doll meant. When I opened the photo book, there was a photo of Beau's birth mom. The actress doll was amazingly similar to the birth mom's image. I was stunned. The hair, the dress color, shape, collar, and even the pose she was in, was just like the birth mom's photo. Beau had picked a replica of his birth mom out of over 300 objects within minutes of entering our therapeutic space. He had chosen the replica of his birth mother from the day he last saw her, from that day when he was two weeks old. The next photo showed the four parents with the adoption lawyer as they completed their arrangement. Everyone was smiling, except Beau.

Beau portrayed many stories and patterns and taught me a

great deal about prenatal and neonatal memory, traumatic impacts, and the expressions of them. For example, he repeated a particular sequence over and over again. He would ask for a doll and then throw it on the floor. When his mother would say, "I want this baby" and try to pick it up, he would become agitated, reach for the baby and try to throw it away saying, "No, you don't want that baby." This appeared to be a belief he carried about himself and his sense of being thrown away and being unwanted based on his earlier experience.

Sometimes, Beau would choke a baby against the wall repeatedly. Later, the birth mom confirmed that when she told the birth father she was pregnant, he was so angry, he had pushed her against the wall and choked her.

Often young children showed me experiences from prenatal life. The perspective varied in the stories. In the choking incident portrayal, Beau had taken the biological father's perspective. Other times, children would act out something that happened to the mother as they identified with her. But children also portrayed their own perspective in relationship to events and parent's perspectives. The following story tells a boy's story about what he needed to have heard from his own perspective.

Four-year-old Stevie announced, "Next time we play with these!" as he pointed to a distinct outdoor sand tray scene in my office. Two weeks later, he marched in and put the outdoor scene up high on top of a folded futon. He would not tell his mother and me the story, we had to guess it. When we failed to understand it's meaning, he took a bat and destroyed the scene. Then he rebuilt it. I started asking his mom when they might have been at an outdoor scene like the one portrayed—as a child, as an infant? The mom paused, "I don't think it could be it, but when I was five months pregnant with him, I had a trip to a place like that and it was a very stressful weekend." Bingo—he smiled. Over the next thirty minutes he brought out more objects to add to the scene. We were to guess each time what scenario he was depicting.

He essentially told several specific elements of the weekend's events in sequence! Each piece was something that was emotionally charged and had held the mother's intense focus during the stressful trip. He was clearly upset about it all. During the session, his mother got that he was very "there" during this intense weekend experience. She realized she had been so stressed and focused on meeting the crises that she had not considered that Stevie, at five months in utero, could be consciously aware of the events and her stressful responses to them, or could be directly affected by them. After she told him how sorry she was and empathized with how hard it must have been, he acted proudly complete with the matter.

The way Stevie told his story is representative of hundreds of stories babies and children have told over the years in my presence. I do not think Stevie could have verbalized the story in sequence, but as we were *in it* he rather *organically* came up with the next piece. What I experienced with children was their ability to portray their memories and stories through movement, activities, symbolic play, gestures, conversation, somatic expressions, and states of being. Often I tried to explain to others the sense of these sessions; I would say that when I became receptive to their material during a session and we were flowing in it, it felt as if we stepped into the Aboriginal Dreamtime of *intuitive being*.

These examples have depicted children initiating a story or

gesture in reference to something that happened. One more child's story comes to mind, that of a six-year-old boy, Terry, who came in with his parents. Utilizing my props, I invited him to make up a game. He put his mom and me behind a futon on end as a wall and his dad across the room on all fours. He got more and more excited as he created the game. He was to ride his father across the room and charge the fort, busting the wall down and then we would all tumble on the floor together. He loved it and wanted to do it again and again. As he charged the fort one last time, he triumphantly added, "Ready or not, here we come!" What was this story about? I knew he was having problems at school. The teacher would ask him to do a task and he would not even try to do it, even though he was capable of it. So there was something about initiation or an issue at the beginning of the sequence at school.

During the session I then asked his parents about his conception—the beginning of things. They paused and then turned wide-eyed. He was conceived even though they had been using a diaphragm and had not wanted another child—"ready or not here I come!" He had just portrayed the story of his conception. I wondered if the "not trying" at school was related to this potentially conflicted beginning. I asked them to talk about how they felt when they found out they were pregnant. They were hesitant out of wanting to protect him from the information. Yet I had already seen how much healing could happen when the truth of some early experience was acknowledged with care. As his mother said hesitantly, "We were a little upset," Terry interrupted loudly, "You were mad!"

When I asked his mother if she was really *that* mad, she shyly nodded yes. The parents then explained hesitantly that they were very angry about being pregnant. It had caused a major rift between them that lasted the entire pregnancy. As they began talking, Terry crawled away and sobbed. His parents then understood that some part of him knew and had felt this conflict and rejection. They were moved to tears and began to tell him how sorry they were, that when he was born, they fell in love with him. (When he was born, he was blue and not breathing. It was at that pivotal moment that they discovered how much they wanted him.)

As his parents were saying how sorry they were and telling him things they loved about him, he slowly crawled to his mother's lap and let her stroke his head. The following session, the mother told me that was the first time he had let her cuddle him and that during the week he had asked her to tuck him into bed, which he had never done before. This story portrays experiences from conception, discovery, and prenatal life that were apparently currently affecting him in his relationship with his mother and his work at school.

We know in therapeutic work that acknowledging what happened to a person, empathizing and feeling that sense of remorse or sorrow that he or she had experienced the earlier difficulty or trauma, is an important aspect of healing. These stories portray children having their stories from conception, prenatal, birth, and neonatal life validated, acknowledged, and responded to with compassion and empathy. The change in patterns and relational dynamics revealed the therapeutic benefit of working with the unresolved early material. (More clinical baby and children stories are included in works cited by Castellino, Emerson, McCarty, and others listed in the Appendix Bibliography.)

These stories were some of the first in my practice over ten years ago. They represent many more told or portrayed to me.

For the first year or so, I videotaped and transcribed my sessions, recording verbal and non-verbal aspects of their communication, movement patterns, symbolic play, parent-child interactions, and sequencing in order to develop my ability to perceive what they were showing me and what interventions appeared to be effective or not.

The children's integrity of being, the "purity" of their expressions, and their organic, visceral responses seen over and over again demonstrated to me that our earliest experiences during our conception, prenatal life, birth, and neonatal period are a part of our being that deeply shape who we become. I came to understand that children had been telling/portraying/living their stories of these experiences all along. We just didn't have a receptacle to receive them in our biologically based conceptualizations of early experience.

The Question of Our Basic Nature

In 1993, I co-founded BEBA, a non-profit research clinic to develop and study PPN-oriented work with babies and their families with Ray Castellino, D.C. We began to work with families as students videotaped our sessions. We would de-brief the sessions and review the videotapes to better understand what these very young babies were showing us. Many of the constrictive patterns and communications appeared to be associated with stressful or traumatic prenatal and birth experiences. These patterns appeared to be implicit belief patterns that were holistic in nature, having somatic, energetic, emotional, mental, and relational elements. The babies also demonstrated the ability to comprehend complex verbal communication and enter into mutual interactions that went beyond traditionally portrayed abilities. For further discussion and four clinical examples, see my article, *The Power of Beliefs: What Babies are Teaching Us* (2002a) that is included in this book as the Appendix *The Power of Belief.*

In 1999, Marti Glenn approached me to collaborate and join a core team to open Santa Barbara Graduate Institute with the first master's and doctoral degrees in prenatal and perinatal psychology (PPN). I chaired the PPN program and Glenn and I co-authored the PPN degree programs. It was a very exciting endeavor that brought me full circle. For three decades the field of prenatal and perinatal psychology had been like a baby, growing and developing in its womb, as it explored the baby's point of view of early experience.

This growing field was being birthed into the outer world and forming relationships with the other blossoming developments in infant psychology, neuroscience, attachment, parent-infant psychotherapy, and infant development. With these new developments, my dilemma re-emerged. After allowing myself to let go of previous notions of infant development and theory and exploring the PPN perspective for a decade, I was surfacing to reconnect with current infant theory, research, and practice. As I did so, I felt the strain of these two perspectives.

In some ways our findings appear to be bringing us closer and closer together, while on the other hand, deep paradoxes and differences remain. For example, I would sit with Piaget's cognitive development theory and research of object permanence. Then, I would hear another PPN-oriented story, such as the following story related by a mother, Rachel, about her son, Vinnie. After hearing a PPN talk about how conscious babies are at birth, Rachel decided to talk to her three-year-old son about his birth, their separation after birth, and why that had occurred. As she began telling him about the separation, he chimed in, "Yeah, I didn't like that. I didn't think you were going to come back. I didn't know if you were going to come back."

In this conversation, Vinnie very spontaneously and in a matter-of- fact way revealed that he clearly had a sense of himself and of his mother as being a separate person he was in relationship with as a newborn. So, there was the paradox. The Piagetian theory of object permanence suggests the sense of constancy of other is developed over the first 18 months after birth, and yet this three-year-old child's comments demonstrated he had known his mother was gone, that they were separated, he expressed the emotional tones associated with missing her, AND wondered if she were coming back in the future—all as a newborn!

As a side note, at the time of this conversation, Vinnie had been having very uncharacteristically intense "meltdowns" when his mother began leaving him at preschool, his first experience of being separated from her and left in a group situation. What were the words he would say to her in the midst of this? "But, I'll never see you again. You may never come back." It appeared that being left at this group preschool had triggered a traumatic memory from being separated at his birth. After this conversation acknowledging what happened at his birth and his feelings about it, his current separation anxiety response dissipated without further intervention.

Returning to the dilemma then of how to make sense of early development research, clinical findings from these very different understandings became a renewed focus of mine. At the core of the differences appears the question of *our basic nature.*

Are we humans that develop consciousness as our form develops and we experience human life? Or are we sentient consciousness, having a sense of self as we enter form? Could both be true when threaded together in a new way?

I'd like to introduce one more important thread of my personal tapestry that is an integral part of my orientation, my spirituality. I was very religious and passionate about my belief in God during high school. Then one night, classmates were talking about the religions of the world and my bubble of beliefs that my church had instilled in me was burst by the diversity of religious perspectives I was introduced to. I stopped attending church because I questioned what my church portrayed as *the truth*. I spun away from religion until my thirties when, during my seven-year journey in infertility, I ventured into the depths of introspection and searching.

I began reading metaphysically oriented books that were outside traditional religious teachings. I voraciously read and experimented with a wide range of topics under the title of consciousness studies, parapsychology, spirituality, and transpersonal psychology. The commonality in these schools of thought was that they spoke to our spiritual nature, our expanded realms of consciousness, and the continuity of life before, during, and after human existence.

In 1989, I found an avenue that felt like home for my spirituality and I began meditating and working in altered states on a regular basis. I discovered I had a natural ability to go into a variety of altered states (without drugs) and experience different aspects of reality that were "nonphysical" in nature. For the last fourteen years, my spirituality has been a central fulcrum of my life, rich with direct experiences, continued explorations through altered

26

states of consciousness, a deepening relationship with the divine, and greater integration as my way of being.

In 1994, the man I was in love with, Bill, died suddenly in an auto accident. He had been a gifted medium and after his death I began an intensive study of consciousness research pertaining to near-death studies, after-death studies, and communicating and working with those in spirit. Many of the beliefs I grew up with were challenged by my direct experiences during this period. These events and the ensuing experiences broadened my views of the continuity of life beyond body and I was deeply changed in this process. I began seeing correlations and similarities between the two transitions of human life—incarnation and death, and appreciated human life more within the greater continuity of existence.

For a long time I felt a split in myself between my traditional nursing and counseling work and my personal spiritual work. When I began my personal and professional PPN-oriented work, it was incredibly healing as I felt a growing sense of the continuity of self and life re-established within me.

In both my professional and personal spiritual journeys, it seemed I needed to fall away from what I had been taught in order to be open to new possibilities through my own direct experiences within myself and with others. I have now come full circle to create a model that begins to bring the fullness of our spiritual and human natures into early development theory, research, interventions, and infant psychotherapy practices.

Chapter III

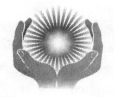

The Broader Context
Moving Towards Integration and Holism

I want to turn our focus from my personal perspective to a broader and more theoretical context in which we can situate the remainder of our discussion. My personal focus on finding an integrated model of early development appears in synchrony with larger movements in physics, worldviews, psychology, and health in which a general progression towards holistic, interconnected, and integrative theories and perspectives has gained considerable momentum in the past twenty years.

From field, holographic, and dynamic systems theories that speak to interconnectedness, to integrative medicine and holistic healing approaches that bring body-mind-spirit together, or to the emerging momentum in qualitative research methodologies, a collective pulse appears to be drawing us into more integrative perspectives and approaches. In psychology, the field of somatic psychology reminds us of the mind-body connection. Transpersonal psychology and consciousness studies expand our definition and study of human nature and human abilities; and integral psychology brings our mind-body-spirit together once again.

Wilber's Integral Approach

At the forefront of this movement is Ken Wilber, identified by some as the most comprehensive philosophical thinker of our time. Over the last twenty-five years Wilber has articulated possibly the most comprehensive science of consciousness and spectrum of human experience to date (see the Appendix Bibliography for a list of Wilber's publications). In volume after volume, he gathers Eastern and Western foundations for consciousness studies and weaves a story of a multifaceted, integrated reality and self that includes consciousness and our core spiritual nature.

His model and framework are intricate and inclusive, thus providing a foundation for viewing the fuller spectrum of human nature, experience, and inquiry. I believe his integral approach provides us with an effective framework of elements and concepts to build an integrated early development model that embraces: (1) our sentient spiritual nature, (2) our prenatal and perinatal experiences, and (3) contemporary early developmental theories.

In this section, let us explore some of the key concepts and perspectives Wilber offers and consider how they may be helpful in holding the synergy of an integrated perspective by using an example from the PPN literature.

In building his Integral Model, Wilber (1998) draws on the virtually universal belief of the *Great Chain of Being* from the major premodern religious traditions.

According to this nearly universal view, reality is a rich tapestry of interwoven levels, reaching from matter to body to mind to soul to spirit. Each senior level "envelops" or "enfolds" its junior dimensions—a series of nests within nests within nests of Being—so that everything and event in the world is interwoven with every other, and all are ultimately enveloped and enfolded by Spirit, by God, by Goddess, by Tao, by Brahman, by the Absolute Self. (p. 6)

In the Great Chain of Being each level is a holon—both a whole in and of itself as well as a part of the next level's holon. Thus, for example, the body is both its own level of reality and a part of the higher, more encompassing level, the mind. Each higher level contains all the elements of the junior level while transcending and adding something new to the previous level. What stands out here is that the physical self is seen as embraced and encompassed by mind-self and they both are a part of soul-self and spirit-self. Soul and Spirit levels of being are seen as more primary than the physical self.

As we will see, this nearly universal perspective that the Spirit and Soul levels of existence are primary and that the spiritual levels encompass and hold the mind and physical levels, not vice versa, is the foundational notion for building an integrated model of early development and understanding the findings in the prenatal and perinatal psychology literature.

In *The Marriage of Sense and Soul: Integrating Science and Religion* (1998), Wilber emphasizes that for most of human existence the Great Chain of Being was the prevalent view of reality until Western civilization during the modern era virtually denied the existence of it. During that time, *scientific materialism* became prominent and:

31

In its place was a "flatland" conception of the universe as composed basically of matter (or matter/energy) and this material universe, including material bodies and material brains, could best be studied by science and science alone. Thus, in the place of the Great Chain reaching from matter to God, there was now matter, period. (p. 10)

Wilber describes three distinct *modes of knowing* that are associated with the levels of the Great Chain of Being. Each mode has its own unique avenue of knowledge and practice to disclose its findings. *Sensory Empiricism* is the mode of knowing associated with the matter and body levels—the physical levels of being. It relies on observation of monological data, e.g., examination of the brain through EEG data. *Mental Empiricism* is the mode of knowing associated with the level of the mind and relies on internal mental experience, such as in phenomenology and hermeneutics in which one dialogues to ascertain knowledge. *Spiritual Empiricism*, the third avenue of knowing, is associated with the higher levels of being of soul and spirit and is gained through direct spiritual experience with the divine and is translogical, transrational, and transmental.

Wilber points out that in the modern era, the higher levels of knowing were collapsed into the sensory empirical, thus reducing what is real to what is known through sensory empiricism. With this collapse, the search for scientific truth was seen as only what could be verified through the senses and observation.

In many ways, our early development perspectives, views of understanding infants, and methods of studying infants portray this Western modern worldview; our focus narrowed to the physical human self. Biology became the foundation, and the levels of mind, and certainly the levels of spirit and soul, were denied or silently unattended. Even today, the vast majority of thousands of articles and texts on early infant development are devoid of any mention of consciousness or spiritual nature, or spiritual and mind planes of reality as aspects of infant experience.

In his writings, Wilber takes us through the progression of the relationship of science and religion from premodern to modern and postmodern eras. He suggests that the challenge for our time is to integrate science and religion. More specifically, it is to integrate science and *authentic spirituality*, that spirituality which is based on direct experience, and spiritual empiricism, rather than religious doctrine. In his extensive writings, he develops his model as a framework to hold the integrity of all three empirical modes of knowing and re-establishes the appropriate parameters for each.

One of Wilber's talents is his ability to assimilate a massive amount of information and find the commonality and patterns within. After gathering thousands of works on every type of human inquiry, Wilber discovered that they could be organized elegantly into three basic perspectives of inquiry: *I*, *We*, and *It*. Each of these perspectives was seen to be a *unique* domain of inquiry and experience.

- The *I* perspective is from the *subjective self's* point of view of aesthetics. It is expressive and its domain is the *beautiful*.

- The *We* perspective speaks to the *intersubjective* domain of the collective interaction and social awareness with its domain, the *good*.

- The *It* perspective focuses on *objective* realities, realities that can be studied and known through empirical and monological means with its domain, the *true*.

33

Each of these domains, Wilber suggests, has its own language, values, focus, and ways of knowing. Wilber took these spheres and created his four-quadrant Integral Model that would hold "a space" for each unique domain. This model has been articulated with effective graphs and charts and woven throughout his various texts, as in *A Theory of Everything* (2000). Virtually every aspect of existence can be included in his model. Table I summarizes the selected elements of his model that we will utilize in building the *Integrated Model* of early development.

Table I
Wilber Integral Model Quadrants

Interior Individual	Exterior Individual
I – Subjective Intentional First person accounts Interpretation Beautiful	**It** – Objective realities Behavioral Third person accounts Truth
Interior Collective	**External Collective**
We – Collective Intersubjective Interpersonal meaning Mutual understanding Worldviews, Culture Morals Goodness	**It** - Objective Functional Fit Interobjective Third person accounts Society Systems theory web Structural/functional Truth

Wilber's Integral Model becomes exquisitely more intricate and developed, but for our purposes it is valuable to simply appreciate that each of these—the three perspectives (*I, We,* and *It*), the four quadrants, and the three ways of knowing—speaks to the *differentiated and unique aspects of inquiry*. In psychology, each of these addresses the differentiated aspects of our inquiry and understanding of human development and human experience.

Wilber points out that many schools in psychology have reduced their focus to only one aspect of psychology, bringing greater understanding in that aspect, but often reducing understanding to their particular focus or aspect of inquiry without integrating information from other schools of thought (2000). For example, a pure behavioral perspective would emphasize the objective external aspects of an issue and leave the interiors unattended. Wilber's Integral Approach attempts to present a framework that would allow the uniqueness of numerous perspectives while integrating them together into one meta-model. In his book *Integral Psychology: Consciousness, Spirit, Psychology, Therapy* (2000) he gathers hundreds of developmental theories and models while presenting an inclusive view of human development and integral psychology.

Wilber's material is invigorating, taking us from the modern era's flatlands into a multifaceted, multidimensional reality that re-infuses our spiritual nature and primary consciousness, re-establishes body-mind-spirit integration, and honors the interior modes of knowing via mind and spiritual empiricism as well as via exterior sensory empiricism. His model and writings contribute greatly with their ability to clarify and embrace the fuller range of early development and PPN by honoring each perspective for its unique contribution.

Wilber repeatedly points out the problem that occurs when any one mode of knowing reduces truth or knowing to its own mode (1998). He also emphasizes that what is true within one mode of knowing will have correlates in the other modes, but warns of the danger that one mode should rest its validity in one of the other modes.

For example, spiritual empiricism is known through the direct experience of the divine and is an interior experience. There is a great deal of research on meditative practices and states of being that speaks to the various levels and types of *interior* experiences of the divine. There is also a body of research that examines the monological correlates of those interior experiences that have mapped out brain wave patterns observed with the various interior meditative experiences.

Wilber cautions us not to use the sensory data to "prove" that the interior states and experiences are real. He suggests that we take great care to honor each distinct mode of knowing and find validity through the process of (1) creating the practice or procedure, "If you want to know about this, then do this practice," (2) have the direct experience and collect the data, and (3) share this with others who have followed the course and see if there is agreement (1998).

Let's examine this issue with the following example. I might say "The experiences reported in meditation of direct experience with the divine are real *because* the EEG readings show us consistent patterns when people are reporting 'XYZ.'" It is very tempting, because I believe we are culturally inclined to give more validity to the sensory mode of "proof" of what is real.

Using our meditation example, Wilber would suggest that although the modes of knowing would find correlates in the other domains, it is still critical to hold each uniquely verifiable within their own domain. In other words, the sensory data will never be able to describe or hold the nature of the internal experience from the meditative experiences. The monological EEG readings can never describe or express a person's interior direct spiritual experience during the meditative state.

Because early development models have thus far been mostly based on the behavioral and sensory empirical infant data and research, with little or no inclusion of the inner realms of mind, soul, and spirit, PPN clinical findings are particularly significant in that they are mapping out the interiors of our earliest experiences and allowing for the rediscovery of our spiritual nature and direct spiritual experience as we begin human life.

Three Modes of Knowing: Dr. Farrant's Conception Journey

The following is a rich example that illustrates several important points. Graham Farrant, an Australian psychiatrist, was one of the pioneers in PPN who unfortunately died without publishing much of his years of clinical PPN findings and experiences (Farrant 1986a/b, Larimore and Farrant, Raymond, 1988).

In the 1970's, Farrant had a "traditional practice" until he was introduced to primal therapy. In one of his own sessions, he found himself exploring the primal terrain of his experiences during the sperm, egg, and conceptus journeys. In 1979, he videotaped himself during a regression therapy session in which he was experiencing what he referred to as the *cellular consciousness* of his conception. He related that during his regression, his body's experience contradicted two currently held medical assumptions. During his primal experience, he related that his mind wanted to use the medical assumptions to discount his own body's experience. For instance, he found himself in his own experience in the journey coming down the fallopian as the fertilized egg and pausing several times to consider whether he really wanted to live.

The following passages about this experience are in his own words from an interview with Steven Raymond in an article for *The Pre-& Peri-natal Psychology News:*

> It felt like a crucial moment of truth, a sensing of the world around, the maternal environment, and the physical, mental and spiritual state of mother as a symbolic partner and whether or not life was to be on this occasion. Now this was my emotional interpretation of my physical experience. However, I was intellectually convinced that the physical reality of the egg was a continuous and progressive rotation and movement down the tube. (Raymond, 1988, p. 5)

In 1983, when the *Miracle of Life* film came out, the sensory visual data demonstrated for the first time that the physical journey of the fertilized egg was as Farrant had experienced it, not as the medical beliefs had suggested. Farrant saw the film and later commented that when the film verified his physical experience, it was "another incredible confirmation of an experience that I had so resisted accepting as true" (p. 6). Farrant expanded upon his interior experience of his pauses in the tube:

> My experience of this float, totally and personally, was that it was a time of spiritual reappraisal, as I mentioned previously. It's another kind of breathing space where the fertilized egg takes stock of its origins, its pre-gamate truth as a spirit or soul. Conception is a trilogy, not a duality. It's a threesome: body, mind and soul; the egg, sperm and soul come together and unite. The pre-conception

consciousness of the gametes has the predominant quality of spirit. Sure it's chemical and biological and physical and it's human, but there's more of a spiritual ethereal quality to it. Once fertilized, there's a kind of looking back to take stock of truth. Jung called it "oceanic bliss," where the human zygote is not attached to the womb wall; it's detached, in the spiritual connotation of detachment. (p. 6)

Farrant related his own inner dialogue about the question of validity of his interior experience.

I originally had the same difficulty as a medically trained scientific person. I wanted double blind studies for "proof," but in psychiatry in general and in regressive therapies in particular, it is extremely difficult to achieve concrete studies. What I have come to rely upon more and more over the years is seeing profound and sustained clinical change in adults who prior to therapy had a multitude of problems. For example, being unable to conceive, or stricken with rheumatoid arthritis or ulcers or other psychosomatic diseases, or psychiatric syndromes that had been previously unresponsive to medication or psychotherapy. In cases such as these, when memories of conception were achieved, expressed, relieved and integrated, and there followed a dramatic, sudden and sustained change in personality, behavior and interactive life experiences, it became convincing to me that the experiences relived in therapy must have had some basis in a concrete reality. (p. 6)

When Raymond questioned him concerning the issue of memory versus the possibility of imposed imagination as explanations of their experiences, Farrant replied:

...I believe the reality of conception experiences in therapy because I have been able to identify specific movements of the body, especially the hands, in relation to specific sequential biological phenomena. These are consistently and spontaneously present in different clients who don't know each other. In their regressions they believe they are re-experiencing various aspects of conception, like implantation, or floating in the womb, or descent in the tube, or conception and pre-conception. It is true they may know my paradigm includes conception, but they do not know the various movements that I have previously correlated with different conception memories, and these physical movements come quite spontaneously, even uncontrollably. This is one reason I am convinced that their experiences are memories instead of metaphors.

However, not only have I discerned specific movements associated with specific conception memories, but I have also been able to link various clinical syndromes to the reports of specific therapy experiences within those first ten days between conception and implantation. (p. 7)

This example of Dr. Farrant's experience speaks to several important points. His experience of the conception journey during his primal regressions are steeped in a deep intertwining of all *three types of knowing*, oriented in *spiritual empiricism, mind empiricism*, and *sensory empiricism*. He found observable correlates in terms of the *Miracle of Life* film and movement patterns that corresponded to the content of the experiences. Yet, it was his description of his integrated modes of knowing his interior experience that brought the profundity of the conceptus journey to life.

So much of the PPN-oriented findings from clinical reports from adults and children are from the interior (the upper-left-hand quadrant in Wilber's model), reports on levels of being that appear to intertwine our higher modes of knowing from the soul and spirit levels with our mind and body levels. This is unique, because the vast majority of the early development research and theory comes from sensory empiricism and external observations. Wilber's recommendation to take great care to respect each way of knowing as valid in its domain is important because respecting and understanding the "realness" of the higher modes of knowing in early development is crucial for the integrity of our models.

This section focused on the broader context in which an Integrated Model of early development and experience may be situated. In the modern era, scientific materialism dominated worldviews with the collapse of spiritual and mind empiricism into sensory empiricism. The Western worldview therefore focused on views of reality based on matter and the biological nature of life.

In the postmodern era, Wilber (and others) have suggested that our task is now to restore what was considered nearly the universal view prior to the modern era, that of the Great Chain of Being. This worldview holds that the physical level is but one level encompassed in a tapestry of progressive, interwoven levels reaching from body to mind to soul to spirit, with the spiritual levels as primary. Each level has its own unique mode of knowing and empirical methods. Dr. Farrant's conception journey demonstrates how each way of knowing contributes to our greater understanding of early human experience.

Our Interconnected Universe

Now that we have a broader context and framework in which to place our model, I want to discuss some key concepts and principles related to sensory empiricism in physics to help orient our phenomenological findings and discussion in the next section. The style and tone of this section shifts into more of a presentation of ideas, theories, and information.

Each of these has made me more receptive to new ways of conceiving and perceiving reality, ways of being in the world. The following ideas were thus instrumental to the creation of the proposed Integrated Model of early development. Over the last twenty years, my journey has been a tapestry of: (1) direct experiences that did not fit into the old Newtonian model—not only my experiences with babies, but also much of my spiritual and metaphysical experiences, my experiences in healing, and in ways of proactively creating my life; and (2) reading and exploring theories and findings that not only validated what my direct experiences were revealing, but also offered new perspectives, new ways of conceiving and perceiving, that awakened more expanded possibilities to further explore my direct experience.

The tone and voice of this next section shifts into more of a direct presentation of information. Several important theories and findings from the fields of physics, holographic theory, morphogenetic fields, memory, and continuity of life outside of human existence are highlighted. In the next chapter, we utilize these concepts to build the Integrated Model. The material here is rather dense and may work well as a reference to return to for further consideration.

As we have discussed, prior to the modern era, the holonomic worldview was based on the Great Chain of Being:

> According to this nearly universal view, reality is a rich tapestry of interwoven levels, reaching from matter to body to mind to soul to spirit. Each senior level "envelops" or "enfolds" its junior dimensions—a series of nests within nests within nests of Being—so that every thing and event in the world is interwoven

with every other, and all are ultimately enveloped and enfolded by Spirit, by God, by Goddess, by Tao, by Brahman, by the Absolute Self. (Wilber, 1998, p. 6)

In this view, our spiritual nature was held to be primary and our physical existence was held within it. During the modern era, scientific materialism became the dominant worldview and Newtonian physics came to view the world mechanistically. For the first time, the manifest physical world of matter was considered the fundamental reality. According to Newtonian physics, matter could be reduced to discrete separate units, with the whole being the sum of its parts, and best understood by objective sensory measurements. The world was viewed as an objective reality to which we were separate observers.

Time and space were absolute and everything could be explained by reference to their causes and observations. Space was considered to be empty and was discounted even in mathematical calculations as inconsequential. The impact of this worldview pervaded not only physics, but also every area of inquiry including psychology, early development, and, as Larry Dossey, M.D., discusses, medicine (1999). For those of us living in the 20th century, this view has been the foundation of how we perceive and conceive what is real and even how we live day-to-day in the world.

However, this view of reality unraveled during the 20th century as physicists began disproving many of its basic tenets. By contrast, the new physicists began describing the universe not as a machine, but rather as a *living ever-evolving organism, holographic and holonomic in nature.* In an interview, quantum physicist David Bohm characterized the nature of the universe as, "the whole is present in each part, in each level of existence. The living reality, which is total and unbroken and undivided, is in everything" (Wilber, 1982, p. 192). He described existence as the universal unbroken wholeness in perpetual dynamic flux and ever-changing movement.

Physicists discovered matter was not the fundamental unit with empty space surrounding it. As they broke matter into smaller and smaller units, it reached a point where it no longer possessed any dimension at all. What used to be considered empty space between matter was actually found to be an infinite sea of connected non-dimensional fields of waves of energy. The fabric of this sea is called zero-point energy. As McTaggart explains in *The Field: The Quest for the Secret Force of the Universe,*

> The zero-point energy was the energy present in the emptiest state of space at the lowest possible energy, out of which no more energy could be removed—the closest that motion of subatomic matter ever gets to zero. (2002, p. 20)
>
> The existence of the Zero Point Field implied that all matter in the universe was interconnected by waves, which are spread out through time and space and can carry on to infinity, tying one part of the universe to every other. (2002, p. 24)

The following two examples give us a sense of the magnitude of the energy held in this zero-point energy in space. Physicist Richard Feyman relates, "The energy in one cubic matter of space is enough to boil all the oceans of the world" (2002, p. 24). Talbot writes, "When physicists calculate the minimum amount of energy a wave can possess, they find that every cubic centimeter of empty space contains more energy than the total energy of all the matter in the known!" (1991, p. 51). Thus, space was not only found not to be empty, but also held a magnitude of energy that far exceeded the energy in our world of matter!

Bohm called this order of the universe the *implicit order*. The properties of this order were quite different from those explained by Newtonian principles. The implicit order, not having location or space, is non-local, non-linear, and contains infinite possibilities and energy. Its nature is hidden, unseen, unmanifested, and primary. Existence in the implicit order is enfolded.

Bohm calls the three-dimensional physical world of matter the *explicit order* and suggests that the implicit unfolds in the explicit order. In laboratory experiments, energy was seen to function as waves of energy in the implicit order, and to function as particles when observed by three-dimensional observation methods. In other words, before being observed, energy in the enfolded implicit order functioned as a wave of infinite, unbroken, continuous energy. When observed, it would collapse into a particle in the three-dimensional explicit order, appearing in a specific time and space.

When considering the whole and the interaction between the implicit and explicit order of existence, existence could be seen as a continuous unbroken dance between the implicit and explicit, the hidden All-That-Is implicit order of the universe and our manifest physical explicit order of the universe in an ever-evolving relationship of enfolding and unfolding experience. Bohm states:

> ...empty space has all this energy and matter is a slight increase of the energy, and therefore matter is like a small ripple of this tremendous ocean of energy, having some relative stability, and being manifest. Now, therefore my suggestion is that this implicate order implies a reality immensely beyond what we call matter. Matter itself is merely a ripple in this background. ...And the ocean of energy is not primarily in space or time at all. ...It's primarily in the implicate order. (Wilber, 1982, p. 56)

45

Scientist Mae-Wan Ho, in her article "The Entangled Universe," discusses these concepts in terms of how we view organisms and specifically human beings. Ho suggests:

> Think of each organism as an entity that is not really confined within the solid body we see. The visible body just happens to be when the wave function of the organism is most dense. Invisible quantum waves are spreading out from each one of us and permeating into all other organism.... Each of us has the waves of every other organism entangled within our own make-up... each of us is supported and constituted, ultimately, by all there is in the universe. (2000, p. 23)

One of the most stunning findings and principles of quantum physics is non-locality. In her article, Ho describes the experimental findings that led to understanding non-local entanglement:

> The experiment consists of elementary particles that are prepared in pairs and are allowed to move apart in opposite directions. According to quantum theory, if we measure a property of one of the particles in the pair, such as spin, the other particle would have a correlated property... *no matter how far apart the particles* are when the measurements are made. The results cannot be explained by a signal being sent from one particle and measured by the other. Such a signal if it exists, would have to take no time at all to travel, which is considered impossible in classical physics. The conclusion that has to be drawn is that the effect of measurement (the collapse of the wave function) of one particle is somehow instantaneously communicated to the other one. Before measurement, neither particle actually had the definite property, and the separated particles comprised a *single coherent system*. (2000, pp. 21-22)

Thus, once related or in contact with each other, no matter

how far apart in terms of distance, the particles had the ability to instantaneously influence one another. Think of the myriad implications of this with parents and their children. In Newtonian physics, the whole was seen as the sum of its parts. Now not only was the whole appreciated as more than the sum of its part, the whole was seen to hold the organizing principle for its components!

The Holographic Paradigm

When hearing the word hologram, many of us conjure up fond memories of holographic images from our favorite sci-fi movies; for me, that is Princess Leah's projected three-dimensional image in the movie *Star Wars*. The holographic paradigm suggests our whole universe is holographic in nature, that organisms are holographic, and that our human brains function holographically as well.

In the early 1990s, I read Michael Talbot's book *The Holographic Universe*, and was quite affected by it. Soon thereafter I attended several *Holographic Repatterning* workshops, a system of healing that incorporates the principles of this paradigm. The work was powerful, effective, and brought to life so much of what the holographic theory held. I also trained with Frankyn Sills who incorporated the holographic understanding into his biodynamic craniosacral training, which became a core foundation in my PPN-oriented work. Thus, for me, it has become a foundational framework, both in theory and in practice.

Talbot describes the photographic holographic process that illustrates the holographic concepts and principles:

> A hologram is produced when a single laser light is split into two separate beams. The first beam is bounced off the object to

be photographed, in this case an apple. Then the second beam is allowed to collide with the reflected light of the first, and the resulting interference pattern is recorded on film.

To the naked eye the image on the film looks nothing at all like the object photographed. In fact, it even looks a little like the concentric rings that form when a handful of pebbles is tossed into a pond. But as soon as another laser beam (or in some instances just a bright light source) is shined through the film, a three-dimensional image of the original object reappears. (1991, pp. 14-15)

So a photographic hologram begins as one beam of light and is split into two beams of light. One remains in its original form and is focused on the photographic plate. The other beam goes out and experiences a three-dimensional object (let's say a red rose); it has experience with explicit matter in other words. The two beams of light converge on the photographic plate and create on the plate what look to the human eye like concentric circles (similar to the implicit order interference patterns as an interacting sea of energy waves) and in these, information of *two beams in relationship* (entangled) are held. When a light is shined on the plate, the encoded information from the plate produces the holographic image of the three-dimensional object photographed behind or beyond the plate. So the plate looks like concentric circles, yet when a light is shined on it, the three-dimensional holographic red rose appears in the space beyond it.

Holograms have the capacity to store incredibly large amounts of information. Also, when any fragment of the hologram (the photographic plate) is illuminated, the whole holographic image is re-created, not just the fragment. Thus, in every part, the integrity of the whole is enfolded and, when illuminated, the whole is unfolded, not just the isolated fragment.

In his book *Craniosacral Biodynamics, Vol. I* (2001), Franklyn Sills incorporates the holographic paradigm and holographic human body understandings. In doing so, he articulates another important property of holograms:

> In the absence of the reference beam, an astounding thing occurs. What comes out the other side is chaos. There is no clarity, no coherent image, no order, and no integration. The reference beam, that pure source of light, is essential to maintain order and cohesion. This analogy has vast repercussions in the understanding of all healing work. It is the reference beam that maintains order and allows coherency and integration of function. (p. 42)

The photographic hologram helps us grasp the basic holographic process and principles. Scientists are exploring the holographic processes at various levels of existence—from levels that include the quantum, subatomic, molecular, cellular, organism, and human body and brain. Although fascinating and very relevant, the discussion of these can easily get quite intricate and beyond our focus here. Therefore, I want to just touch on them here and refer you to the Appendix Bibliography for further reading on this vital topic.

Mae-Wan Ho discusses the holographic nature of organisms and suggests that, "The coherence of the organism is maintained through quantum processes that enable instantaneous intercommunication to occur and that memory is distributed over the entire liquid crystalline continuum of the body which serves as a holographic medium" (2003, p. 197).

She discusses the qualities of the liquid crystalline that serve as the holographic medium support:

> ...The activities of the organism are fully coordinated in a continuum from the macroscopic to the molecular. The organism is coherent beyond our wildest dreams. Every part is in communication with every other part through a dynamic, tunable, responsive, liquid crystalline medium that pervades the whole body, from organs and tissues to the interior of every cell. Liquid crystallinity gives organisms their characteristic flexibility, exquisite sensitivity, and responsiveness, thus optimizing the rapid intercommunication that enables the organism to function as a coherent whole. (2000, p. 20)

In this passage, Ho is discussing the holographic nature of organisms. In *Nature's Mind: The Quantum Hologram* (2003), Edgar Mitchell, an Apollo 14 astronaut and the founder of the Institute for Noetic Sciences, discusses holographic findings at several levels. At the quantum level (implicate order), he describes the quantum hologram as a *fundamental non-local information carrier*. A helpful analogy is that the quantum hologram is to matter as the mind is to the brain. Citing various sources of research, Mitchell suggests that the:

> Information carried by the quantum hologram encodes the complete event history of the object with respect to its three-dimensional environment. It evolves over time to provide an encoded non-local record of the "experience" of the object in the four-dimensional space/time of the object as to its journey in space/time and the quantum states visited.

One of the profound implications of this is that the quantum hologram has the entire history of each object encoded in the implicate order, and therefore each human individual, including our experiences at all levels of our being. Returning to Wilber's terms, the quantum hologram then would have encoded information of our full range of sensory, mental, and spiritual levels of experiences.

Mitchell believes the quantum hologram can explain Rupert Sheldrake's theory of *morphic resonance*. Schwartz and Russek (1999) describe Sheldrake's thesis as follows:

> Sheldrake's thesis is that objects come into being (atom, cells, organs) not only because of information inside them, such as the genetic code, but because of information and energy outside, called "fields" in physics. ...He proposed that this morphic field grew with experience; meaning, each time an object came into existence, it added its form information to the overall morphic field. Hence the field was continuously evolving, accumulating information with each new thing. With continued replication, the birth of atoms, crystals, cells or organisms should be easier to occur over time.... What Sheldrake proposed was that the information was stored everywhere, equally, and this storage transcended space and time. (pp. 123-124)

Jean Houston, scholar and researcher in understanding and tapping latent human abilities, in her article "Reality and How It Works," articulates one of the important implications of Sheldrake's theory nicely:

> ...we are all connected through what Sheldrake calls "morphogenetic fields," organizing templates weaving through time and space, which hold the patterns for all structures, but which can be changed according to our changing thoughts and actions. Thus the more an event, pattern of behavior, or skill is duplicated, the more powerful its morphogenetic field becomes.

> Sheldrake states the very basis of paradigm shift: Things are as they are because they were as they were. The laws of nature are not absolutes, rather they are accumulations of habits…. Laws change, habits dissolve, new forms and functions emerge whenever an individual or a society learns a new behavior. (2004, p. 1)

In *The Biology of Transcendence* (2002), Joseph Chilton Pearce discusses morphogenetic fields in terms of the untapped ability of humans to access the infinite amount of information available in these non-local morphogenetic fields. He gives the example of the phenomena of individuals with savant syndrome. These individuals with IQ's of about 25 experience great difficulty functioning in the world, yet are able to access certain areas of knowledge, such as mathematics, and retrieve fantastical information that is beyond what we conceive possible. It is now believed that they are accessing these morphogenetic fields of information in the quantum hologram.

Mitchell suggests that the evolutionary process is guided at the various levels by the non-local quantum hologram and thus the non–local morphogenetic fields. The implication here is that the quantum hologram contains the entire history of our universe and every aspect of it and is theoretically accessible to us.

In their book *The Living Energy Universe: A Fundamental Discovery that Transforms Science & Medicine* (1999), Gary Schwartz and Linda Russek lay out their theory of the "Universal Living Memory." They systematically build the case that every level of existence functions as a dynamic system, in ever-evolving feedback loops of exchanging energy and information. Schwartz and Russek explain:

> The universal living memory process—an expression of evolution in time—is a systemic potential in all systems of

52

recursive/circulating A's and B's.

A's and B's can even be two pendulum clocks on a wall. When set into motion, they will engage in spontaneous resonance, revising their inter-clock relationship, and emerging into a remembered synchrony of swings. The clocks will, so to speak, "self-organize" and become a two-clock, self-revised system. They will ultimately beat as one. (p. 68)

Thus as A and B interact they are forming an A-B system and they "accrue integrative systemic memories," each affected not only by the other, but also by the accrued integrative systemic memories. Their book is a fascinating journey in the evolution of their premise, which weaves findings in biology, morphogenetic field theory, physics, homeopathy, transplant patient experience, after-life existence and communication, and paranormal experiences, such as remote viewing, that are congruent with their theory.

In grappling with the issue of the plausibility of out-of-body consciousness and survival of consciousness after death, they suggest that if everything is ultimately information and energy as quantum physics suggests, and "Information refers to pattern, form, structure. Energy refers to force and power, the capacity to do work and overcome resistance. Energy does the work of information. ...Could it be that soul is to spirit as information is to energy" (p. 101)? They build the case that these dynamic ever-evolving circular feedback loops occur at every level of existence. In essence, they suggest everything at every level of existence is alive, remembers, and evolves, implying that memory (stored information and energy) occurs in the implicit and explicit orders, and between these two orders, and that memory is not dependent on or limited to our physical world.

In his next book, *The Afterlife Experiments: Breakthrough Scientific Evidence of Life after Death* (2002), Schwartz describes his research on contact with individuals after they have died examined under controlled conditions. The evidence is compelling. Thus, in one book, he and Russek address the dynamic feedback process by which memory is theoretically possible in the non-local realms as well as in the physical one. In his next book, Schwartz examines the phenomena of existence and the ability to communicate (receive and send information) with individuals who are no longer in the physical realm. He thus suggests the existence of a sense of individual self after death in which individuals who have "died" have memory of their human life and have the ability to communicate with individuals in the physical world. On the receiver end of the communication, he is also suggesting his research demonstrates the ability of humans to receive information from individuals from the non-local realm. (For other readings in this area see the Appendix Bibliography.)

Mitchell describes the human brain as a quantum brain that utilizes both non-local and space/time information and argues that *both* are necessary for perception of three-dimensional objects. He cites Marcer and Schempp's (1997, 1998) description of the brain as a "massive parallel quantum processor" with the capacity to decode the information accessed.

Remember that the photographic holographic image needs to have both beams projected onto the plate—the beam that experiences the three-dimensional object and the beam of pure light—to be successfully created. Mitchell explains what is thought to be necessary for a three-dimensional reality to be perceived as it is and where it is:

It is not sufficient for the incoming electromagnetic illumination (or acoustic signal) carrying object information to present to the brain a wave front in the manner presented to a flat photographic plate. Rather, a virtual signal as mapped by the phase conjugative or quantum holographic formalism is required to decode the information in order for perception and cognition to exist as we experience it in three-dimensional reality. The percipient and the source of information are in a resonant relationship for the information to be accurately perceived.

Thus, we do not directly perceive a physical object, we receive physical and quantum information about that object and our system decodes that into a perception of the three-dimensional reality of that object. In order for us to perceive something as real in our three-dimensional world, we must be resonant with the event or object we are perceiving. We must be "in phase" (the technical term is phase-conjugate-adaptive-resonance or pcar).

The movie *Field of Dreams* offers a non-technical example that illustrates this phenomenon well. In the movie, a couple builds a baseball field and players from what might be called the "non-local implicit world" come to play on their field. They perceive them as real. The brother-in-law does not perceive the players on the field. He does not believe it is possible, and he does not perceive they are there until a pivotal moment at which point he begins to see them. We could postulate that the brother was not "in phase" or in resonance with the reality and therefore did not perceive them. Once the shift had occurred, he perceived the ballplayers as the rest of those present did.

Mitchell postulates that intuitive information, what he calls *intuitive perception*, occurs when a perceiver is in phase with the object or entity associated with the quantum hologram. This speaks to perception at a non-local level. Mitchell references the extraordinary findings reported by Dean Radin in *The Conscious Universe: The Scientific Truth of Psychic Phenomena* (1997). Radin provides meta-analysis of hundreds of trials that demonstrate perception of non-local information. Remote viewing, telepathy, clairvoyance, and intuition are examples of the types of non-local perception demonstrated in which the person is receiving information. In other experiments, individuals and groups of individuals are senders of information locally.

Strong evidence demonstrates our ability to influence matter, inanimate objects and machines as well as animate receivers, including other human beings, at a distance with the use of our *attention and intention*. An example of this type of non-local influence is intentional distant healing phenomenon. What is striking about non-local events is that by their very nature they are not dependent on or within our usual time/space constraints. Therefore, their impact does not dissipate over distance and occurs instantaneously. This makes them distinctly different from energetic interactions in which there is a thermodynamic transfer of energy that does take time and dissipates with distance.

Mitchell points out that most humans do not bring non-local information to consciousness when functioning day-to-day. Although some people appear to be psychically or intuitively sensitive to this order of information, Mitchell suggests that:

> It takes training as provided by many of the esoteric traditions and/or certain naturally sensitive individuals to routinely perceive the non-local holographic information associated with a particular object. There is massive evidence to suggest, however, that the

brain has these latter capabilities at birth. Suppression by cultural conditioning in childhood and subsequent lack of practice cause the natural ability of conscious, intuitive perceptions to atrophy. Particularly in western tradition, educational interest has been on the left brain, rational functions rather than on the right, intuitive function. However, mystic adepts and natural psychics routinely demonstrate that non-local information is perceptible from physical objects by focusing attention, quieting the left brain and allowing intuitive perceptions to appear. The fact that with training and practice, individuals can recover, deepen and label their individual cognitive access to intuitive, non-local information demonstrates that learning is taking place with the whole brain itself and involves enhanced coherence and coordination between the hemispheres.

Psychic phenomena, meditative spiritual experiences, and non-ordinary states of consciousness all appear to be associated with tapping non-local time/space dimensions of our physical world.

My last quote from Mitchell's article is very poignant for our discussion:

> …the quantum hologram can properly be labeled as "nature's mind" and that the intuitive function we label in humans as the "sixth sense" should properly be called the "first sense." The perception of non-local information certainly preceded and helped to shape, through learning feedback, the sensory systems that evolved in planetary environments, and which we currently label as the five normal senses.

Although I find this arena of discussion a fascinating one, for our purposes here, I have just highlighted a few points to give us some sense of how much our worldviews and scientific findings regarding the nature of our reality have changed dramatically over the last few decades—moving from a Newtonian framework into a view of our physical existence situated within the quantum hologram, a self-organizing, learning, interactive, interconnected, evolving whole; a reality in which the quantum realms of the enfolded implicit realms, outside of time and space, are an essential and primary order of our universe.

Now let us bring this discussion of physics into Wilber's four-quadrant model as portrayed in Table I. Wilber's model is inclusive of all arenas of inquiry and understandings of reality and human existence. Physics is a field of inquiry that focuses on the objective external world of *IT*. It relies on sensory empiricism's observation of the physical objective world and mental empiricism (mathematics). In the next section, I return to our exploration of early development in which there is a large emphasis on the interior exploration of existence. Thus, with Wilber's framework and these current understandings in mind, let us turn now to the phenomenological experiences relevant to the creation of an integrated model of early experience.

Chapter IV

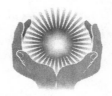

Building the Integrated Model
Of Early Development

Coming to terms with the differences between traditional early development views based on a biological understanding of early development and views from prenatal and perinatal psychology research and my work with babies and children has been a compelling motivation in this process. Worldviews, conceptualizations, research methodologies, clinical applications, and language expressed in the early development and PPN literatures can vary so greatly that I feel like I could be talking about different planets or species. At other times, I find recent thought and research bringing the perspectives closer and closer, bridging our understandings.

In the last decade, with the help of brain imaging technology, for example, our understanding of early infancy has been transformed. Recent work in affective neurosciences and attachment theories has given us a stunning appreciation of the importance of our early experience and the essential role of our relationship with mother (caretaker) in our healthy development. Our early experiences are seen as architects of our growing brain and body's structure that create a lasting blueprint.

In early development literature, models of nonlinear dynamic systems, self-organization, and complexity theory are replacing more fragmented models of early development. In Alan Fogel's foreword to Lewis and Granic's *Emotion, Development, and Self-Organization: Dynamic Systems Approaches to Emotional Development*, he describes *dynamic systems models* as "…characterized by self-organization through iterative feedback processes that afford the possibility of both stability and change, dynamic pattern formation and emergent innovation, order and chaos, determinism and indeterminism" (2000, p. xi).

Lewis and Granic introduce the orientation of the self-organization as referring to the:

> …emergence of order from disorder, and in particular the emergence of coherent, higher-order forms from the interactions of many lower-order components" and "models of self-organization describe the emergence of order, coherence, organized complexity, and true novelty in all natural systems. (p. 9)

Allan Schore, Dan Siegel, Edward Tronick and others have revolutionized understandings of early human development by articulating the intricate dyadic self-organization system necessary for healthy early development. (For future readings in this arena, see the Appendix Bibliography.) Thus so much of the older Newtonian styled models are now seen to have lost their ability to explain and accurately describe early development. These newer models are reflective of the movement towards a *higher order of integration and complexity in the understanding of the whole self in relationship.*

So, in building an integrated model of early development, there is a great deal to bring to the table from the early development communities. Many of our findings from prenatal and perinatal oriented clinical work, are consistent with the newer early development findings and perspectives.

Many needs identified in early development literature as important for healthy development and as profoundly and positively influencing the architecture of the infant's brain and system are considered in the PPN literature to be true for what is optimal from the beginning of life, from conception. I believe the new frontier in early development, where the next level of understanding of optimal growth and development is now, entails taking these new findings and bringing them into a larger context that is situated in the mind-soul-spirit levels of Self and Reality.

In so many other arenas of inquiry that speak to spiritual and mental empiricism and that investigate the levels of mind-soul-spirit, such as in transpersonal psychology, consciousness studies, meditation practices, spirituality, near-death research, human intention, distant healing, and much more, we find evidence and support for our *multidimensional nature* that is not limited to the laws of nature in the three-dimensional physical world.

In the last decade these arenas of inquiry and findings have transformed views of self, reality, and healing as mentioned in Chapter III, resulting in a growing appreciation of a whole new spectrum of human potential that has remained untapped. Yet there is a frontier that is new even to the communities exploring our transcendent/transpersonal/non-local nature. Most of the work

61

has focused on work with transpersonal capacities during adulthood and the transcendent existence as evidenced in near-death or after-death research. I find that when I mention PPN clinical findings that substantiate research in these fields, many listeners initially find it difficult to even imagine the notion of our transcendental nature and our capacities as we come into embodiment.

The acceptance of a more integrated view of self and reality in mainstream thought is an important step towards deepening understanding of human development at the critical, earliest stages. Prenatal and perinatal clinical findings and what babies are teaching us in particular can illuminate the bridge between our various perspectives on early development and provide a common ground for the integration of fields of knowledge related to the beginning of our life cycles. This discussion will unfold in the years to come.

Our Fundamental Transcendent Nature

The most important ground upon which to build the Integrated Model is the fundamental wisdom that *our primary nature is as conscious, sentient, non-physical beings that exist prior to and beyond physical human existence.* Many traditions incorporate the basic holonomic Great Chain of Being into their models, viewing the spirit level or non-physical reality of existence as primary. Within these traditions, the *involutionary* process is viewed as a moving away from Source and into form, a process in which consciousness is seen to precipitate from the non-physical realms of reality that exist outside of time/space into the three-dimensional reality of existence. Our biological human self is seen as an explicit expression of our more fundamental implicit spiritual self.

Not only do PPN clinical findings consistently portray this sentient nature from the beginning of life, they also reveal why it is so crucial to reintegrate our sentient spiritual nature into our theories, research, and practices. The most powerful themes echoed throughout the PPN literature are the myriad unfortunate-to-tragic repercussions from the denial or lack of understanding of our sentient spiritual nature and our sensitive-aware human nature.

Throughout the modern era, Western society increasingly focused on the "sciences" and lost touch with the primary sentient spiritual nature of humanity that is so essential to an accurate understanding of the beginning of human life. This emphasis on empirical, scientific knowledge created an unnatural split in the innate self by diminishing our ability to tap the multidimensional self and its attendant capacities, and by creating traumatic imprinting by our ensuing "scientific" practices.

In the PPN clinical reports of treating adults, children, and babies over the last thirty years through a variety of therapeutic approaches, we see unfortunate to tragic repercussions from the lack of recognition that the baby is sentient–aware, has memory, and is profoundly affected by experiences from the beginning of life. With this, we are witnessing a significant *spectrum of unmet needs* in the baby from the beginning of life.

The PPN clinical reports consistently reveal harmful lifelong effects from Western biologically based medical interventions during conception, prenatal care, birth, and the neonatal period when carried out without the understanding and inclusion of our sentient nature and early needs. (See the Appendix Bibliography for extensive list of references in this arena.) Thirdly, we see that such procedures have resulted in a rupture with our innate instincts and natural attunement with babies as parents, caregivers, and professionals.

Generation after generation, attunement, instincts, and innate knowledge of our nature and of holding the vision of the whole self from the beginning of life has been disrupted. This unnatural split or dissociation became embedded in our subconscious, DNA, and collective morphogenetic fields. It has been passed on and maintained through resulting childrearing practices and medical care that recapitulate and perpetuate the schism in our culture.

When I look back over how I was taught in the 1970's and how I taught others to care for babies being born, what I believed to be "in the best interest of the child," I am saddened that I was perpetuating "unnatural" obstetric practices. At the time, and because of my own birth in which I was separated from my mother, separating mothers and babies seemed natural—"that's how the story goes." Yet, once I re-connected with my birth experiences, worked with others, and read the PPN clinical reports, I felt like I regained my innate knowing and saw how unnatural and disruptive this practice was. For me, the "modern medicine" practice of separating mothers and babies at birth exemplifies the depth of our split from our innate knowing and attunements with babies.

Although many developed societies have seen advancements in understandings of the exterior physical worlds and systems, an appreciation for innate wisdom, interior knowledge, and humans' integrated spiritual nature has greatly diminished. As many authors in the PPN literature have articulated, our birth and parenting practices have become centered on a technological medical model that emphasizes the physical aspects of the birth process and failed to recognize its sentient spiritual nature.

In *The Scientification of Love,* obstetrician Michel Odent cites an ethnological review of historically and geographically diverse cultures that found: "The greater the need to develop aggression and the ability to destroy life, the more intrusive the ritual and cultural beliefs in the period around birth have become" (1999, p. 26). He writes that cultures in which the fundamental innate need for mother and baby to be uninterrupted in their intricate dance during the transition of birth was respected were found to be the same cultures that valued nonaggressive communal living and sought to live in harmony with the ecosystem.

This core split is presently appearing in two opposing current trends in the fields related to childbirth and neonatal care: on the one hand there is increased support for the intricate natural process, as evidenced, for example, in the growing number of facilities adopting the Mother-Friendly and Baby-Friendly guidelines for medical care (www.motherfriendly.org and www.babyfriendly. org). At the same time, however, there has also been an increase in medical interventions not only during childbirth, as evidenced with increasing use of epidural anesthesia, inductions, and in cesarean section surgeries; but also in an increase of various high-tech assisted conception procedures.

When we bring our orientation back to the Great Chain of Being, we reestablish ties with our multidimensional nature in which the levels of experience are woven into an integrated self—physical, mind, soul, and spirit. In many indigenous cultures, that knowing has remained an integral part of life, particularly with respect to how indigenous people acknowledge and respect sentient consciousness during conception, pregnancy, and birth.

In 2003, I heard Sobonfu Somé, author of *Welcoming Spirit*

Home: Ancient African Teachings to Celebrate Children and Community (1999), speak. She described several rituals still practiced by her Dagara tribe in West Africa to prepare for and welcome the baby. Listening to her and reading her book was like entering the dreamtime; her message is poetic, nourishing, and deeply touching because it holds the integrity of the whole multidimensional self.

In her tradition, communication with the pre-conceived child in spirit and throughout the pregnancy is an integral aspect of welcoming and nurturing beings as they journey from the spirit world into the physical domain. A high level of instinctual attunement between baby and mother are the norm. A shrine for the baby is kept during the pregnancy so that each community member can come to communicate with the baby, offering their assistance and welcoming them. These rituals honor and support the baby's sacred journey from the unseen into human life by receiving and preparing the infant according to the soul's communication with him or her. Learning of their ways reawakened within me more of my innate wisdom with respect to welcoming the incoming consciousness.

Unfortunately, much of what we have learned in the Western world about our early prenatal and perinatal experiences from the baby's point of view is how disconnected and out of attunement we have become. It calls us to remember.

Our Sentient Nature and the Continuity of Sense of Self

Memories of prenatal and perinatal experiences reported at all ages are consistently imbued with a sense of self that is assumed unquestionably by the person reporting. Along with this sense of

66

self in early experience is the consistently reported innate desire for those around them to recognize and relate to them as sentient conscious beings. This is evident in Emily's statement, cited above, "They don't know I'm a person. I *know* I am." Similarly, Chamberlain shares another patient's report, Deborah's, in which she reports she felt the adults in the delivery room did not understand her true nature:

> ...I saw all these people acting real crazy. That's when I thought I really had a more intelligent mind, because I know what the situation was with me, and they didn't seem to. They seemed to ignore me. They were doing things *to* me, to the *outside* of me. But they acted like that's all there was. When I tried to tell them things, they just wouldn't listen; like that noise wasn't really anything (her voice). It didn't sound too impressive, but it was all I had. It just really felt like I was more intelligent than they were. (1999, p. 90)

In this situation, Deborah felt she knew what was going on, was trying to communicate with the adults present and yet they were not perceiving or meeting her at that level. This is a recurring theme in PPN clinical reports.

Here is one more example of this type of response from a person remembering birth under hypnosis (Wambach, 1979):

> For me, it seemed I was out of the birth canal quickly, as though I were pulled out. As soon as I emerged it was very scary with lots of lights. People were handling me in a very unloving way, very cold emotionally. I was aware of their feelings. They were doing their job and had good intentions. They were just not aware of their own insensibility and how much I could understand. (pp. 131-132)

Given a general culture proclivity toward the physical aspect of reality, it can be difficult to a grasp the meaning of the phrases "sentient nature" or "conscious and aware and communicating meaningfully from the beginning of life." I have given some examples in this book that suggest certain qualities, but let us examine those qualities more systematically here, for they will become the foundation of the Integrated Model proposed here.

Pre-conception Existence

Many researchers and clinicians have articulated findings indicating we have a sentient self *prior to conception*. (See the Appendix Bibliography.) I will highlight just a few examples for our present discussion.

In their 737-page text *Cosmic Cradle*, Carman and Carman describe their ten-year study of the preconception stage of human incarnation. In their research they found over 165 cultures' and religions' reports of preconception experiences. The scope of the study stretched from antiquity to the present and included every inhabited continent. They also interviewed over one hundred people who described memories of pre-conception experiences and who shared stories of pre-conception communication between parent and their future child.

Many of their interviewees describe memories of existence before and during the process of embodiment from conception through birth. For example, Glenn, a retired military officer who shared his memories of life prior to his conception, described details of preparation in the spirit world for his upcoming life, his journey to earth, and the circumstances and setting of his conception that were later reluctantly confirmed by his mother.

Carman and Carman also include narrative accounts from

children. One striking aspect of the children's recollections of their pre-conception experiences is the matter-of-fact nature of their accounts. For them it appears to be a given. For example, in this account a mother shares her three-year-old daughter's account of coming from "Angel Land":

> Anna Grace told me, "I was up in the Land that I came from, Angel Land. I heard dad calling my name, 'Anna Grace,' and I knew it was time for me to come."
>
> What happened was several weeks before our daughter's birth, my husband suggested the name "Anna Grace." I said, "That is a beautiful name."...
>
> Ana Grace lived in England for six weeks before we moved to America. Yet, she told me many times, "I knew about England because when I was in Angel Land and decided to come here, I saw you in England."
>
> Then she often told me, "I do not like it here. It is too hard. I want to go back to Angel Land." (p. 543)

Carman and Carman summarized their findings in what they called *The Principles of the Cosmic Cradle Pre-Conception Paradigm*. They noted that these principles appeared to be *new* only to materialistic thinking modern culture, echoing our theme. Their principles, gleaned from the breadth of perspectives studied, are:

1. Parenthood begins long before sperm unites with egg.
2. Preparation for human life occurs in the womb of the universe, a hidden realm filled with intelligent souls waiting to be born.
3. Our life plan, or cosmic contract, is designed prior to conception.
4. The boundaries of memory transcend our brain. Human

consciousness exists independently of a brain and nervous system, even before the tiny fetus forms.

5. Individuals with gifted awareness are aware of souls seeking birth and remember pre-uterine life.

6. Human life is the coming together of a mother, father, child's soul, and the soul's cosmic contract. (p. 8)

In *Soul Trek: Meeting Our Children on the Way* (1995), Hallett gathered over 180 accounts of preconception and prenatal communication. Here, Hallet shares a conversation with her own child Devin, then three years old:

> We were sitting together on the back porch of our house when he suddenly said, "Mommy, let's go home."
>
> "Where's our home?" I asked.
>
> "Far, far away," said Devin. Pointing upward, he went on: "Up in the Sunny. This is the dirt place. Our home up there." (p. 263)

What is interesting in accounts like these is that not only are the children very matter-of-fact about their early experience, selfhood, and the communication between parent and child preconceptually, but that they associate their real sense of home in the spirit plane, not the human plane, suggesting that they are sensing the primary nature of their spiritual self prior to entering human lives. Also, similar to Anna Grace's comments, pre-conception memories consistently reveal a differentiated conscious, sentient sense of self prior to incarnation that is capable of communicating with those in the physical world, making choices, and of transcendental perception. The memory of these experiences is then brought into awareness during human life.

This sense of differentiated self is also reported during

conception as portrayed in a conception from Linn, Emerson, Linn, and Linn's *Remembering Our Home: Healing Hurt and Receiving Gifts from Conception to Birth* (1999):

> Karen and her daughter and son-in-law, Emily and Steve, were on vacation at a resort. At 3:00 am, Emily and Steve, faces ashen, knocked on Karen's door. They asked Karen if the lights had gone on her room. Karen said "No. What's wrong?" Emily and Steve explained they were awakened by the feeling of someone running across the bed. At first, each thought the other was getting up. At the same moment, all the lights went on in the room. The lights were on separate switches, which meant that someone would have had to go from one switch to another to turn them all on at once. As Karen, Emily, and Steve talked about this, Emily sensed that she had conceived a child. Sure enough Sarah was born nine months later.
>
> Two years after Sarah's birth, the whole family (including Sarah) was together in Karen's kitchen. They recalled the resort vacation. Sarah said, "I remember that place." Her mother said, "How can you remember it? You weren't born yet." Sarah answered, "I was there. Don't you remember? I ran across your bed." No one had ever mentioned to Sarah what had awakened Emily and Steve that evening; yet Sarah apparently remembered her eagerness to be their child. Two years later, Sarah again referred to the evening of her conception. She said, "I was light and I wanted to put more light into the room." (p. 47)

Researchers Stevenson and Bowman have each contributed greatly to the exploration of children's verifiable accounts of past life (see the Appendix Bibliography). Bowman notes that accounts by children have a distinct "matter-of-factness" and demonstrate a sense of continuity of self from other lifetimes to this one (2001).

Stevenson's latest article (2000) relates twenty-two cases in which children's portrayals concerning other lives lived were found to match events in the life of a specific person who had died. He describes how these children's play activities corresponded to specific aspects of previous lives. For example, a child's play activities might correspond to features of the previous life such as vocation, different gender roles related to the sex of the earlier incarnation, and enactment of the mode of death of that person. The style and manner in which children expressed memories and patterns from previous past lives in their play activities is strikingly similar to children's expressions in play and activities of very early prenatal and birth experiences.

Other researchers have documented adults' accounts of other parts of our continuity of self, such as remembered experiences between lives, some describing their planning of their next lifetime (see the Appendix Bibliography.) These are examples that suggest sentient life and sense of self that has continuity from other lifetimes, life in spirit between lifetimes, and sense of self and memory of experiences during the pre-conception period.

Prenatal and Perinatal Experience and Near-Death Experience Reports

Although a thorough review and discussion of the wealth of evidence of the sentient nature during the prenatal and birth time is not possible here, the Appendix Bibliography includes numerous references to further explore this body of evidence. For our purposes here, I would like to discuss three studies that are particularly relevant to current understandings of the whole self in a prenatal and perinatal context.

Wambach (1979) regressed 750 adults under group hypnosis

to describe their experiences prior to this lifetime, during life in the womb, and at birth. During the regression, she posed a large list of specific questions to her subjects, such as: Did you choose to incarnate? Are you aware of the feelings and attitudes of your mother prior to birth? Approximately 40% of those induced completed descriptive written forms that were usable (those alert and clear enough to remember their experience in the regression).

Wambach discovered that 89% of her participants reported two separate and simultaneous sources of awareness. The transcendent voice tended to be devoid of emotion and characterize itself as a disembodied mind hovering around the fetus and mother, being in and out of the fetus. The other vantage point was from the fetal human body, a perspective that was characteristically more visceral and filled with strong emotions. These accounts thus revealed a continual sense of self from two experiential vantage points.

One interesting finding indicated that whereas death in a previous incarnation was reported as pleasant by 90%, being born—beginning the human life cycle—was unhappy and frightening for a majority, with only 26% looking forward to the coming lifetime. Even so, 81% reported that they themselves had chosen to be born. Nearly all of the participants related being aware, presumably telepathically, of their mother's emotions before and during birth. Wambach states that participants were nearly unanimous on one key point:

> They felt that the fetus was not truly a part of their consciousness. They existed, fully conscious, as an entity apart from the fetus. Indeed they frequently reported that the fetal body was confining and restrictive, and that they preferred the freedom of out-of-body existence. It was with much reluctance that many of

them joined their consciousness with the cellular consciousness of the newborn infant.... When all the 750 cases were analyzed, 89% of all subjects responding said that they did not become a part of the fetus or involved with the fetus until after six months gestation. Even then, many subjects reported being "in and out" of the fetal body. They viewed themselves as an adult consciousness relating to the fetal body as a less-developed form of life. (p. 99)

The second study is one that has become a classic in PPN literature, Chamberlain's *Reliability of Birth Memory: Observation from Mother and Child Pairs in Hypnosis* (1986, 1999). Many of the narrative descriptions can be found in his book *Babies Remember Birth* (1988). In his study, Chamberlain hypnotized children (ages 9-23) and their mothers separately and asked them to describe their birth experiences. He then compared the coherency of the child's and mother's memories of the birth. (Pairs chosen included only children who had not been told the details of their birth and who had no conscious memory of their birth.)

Chamberlain found that the independent narratives matched exactly at many points and dovetailed in an interlocking pattern at other points, with the baby having its own experiences. Rarely was there a contradiction and when there was one, it had a different quality, one of fantasy rather than reported memory. He concluded, "The content of birth memories suggests a sophisticated level of physical, mental and emotional consciousness at birth, beyond anything predicted by developmental psychology" (1999, p. 26).

The narratives from the children revealed accurate reports of: time of day, locale, individuals present, verbatim recollections of events outside the womb, paranormal knowledge of unspoken thoughts of others, knowledge of type of delivery, instruments used, room layouts, sequencing of events, and detailed images of outside the womb while baby was still in the womb. Here are two examples of what mothers and children reported during their individual hypnotic sessions concerning situations soon after the birth that demonstrate how literal memories can be:

> **Words and Names.** Child says: "Mother is talking and playing with me. There is a hassle about the name. Mother didn't like V. or G. but daddy did." Mother says, "I'm tickling and playing with her, stroking her. There is a disagreement about the name for the baby. I don't like V. or G. but prefer Mary K. ...
>
> **Reunion.** Mother says: "I pick her up and smell her. I smell her head. I look at her toes and say, 'Oh, God! She has deformed toes!'" Mother then calls the nurse, asks about the toes and receives reassurance that they are normal. Child report: "She's holding me up, looking at me; she's smelling me! And she asked the nurse why my toes were so funny. The nurse said that's just the ways my toes are and that they weren't deformed." (1999, p. 23)

The third study speaks deeply to me. Over the years of exploration, I read and studied research from various points in the continuity of life and collected works on near-death, after-death, out-of-body, reports after life, between lives, and those coming into life, and our abilities and capacities that utilize our non-local nature, from a variety of types of sources. I would look for similarities in reports from many sources of the quality of our experiences and sense of self in various states—those associated with human life, but also those associated with life outside of the three-dimensional physical world of time and space. (Although a fuller discussion of this area is beyond the scope of this work, I have included a sizable portion of these references in the Appendix Bibliography.)

In my workshops, participants would occasionally have a glazed expression when I mentioned the transcendent nature of our prenatal and birth experience memories. It was hard for them to grasp how memories of and reactions to events and the emotional experience of mother could be possible without a developed brain.

Often I would turn our discussion to a more familiar field to many, that of near-death experiences. When we listed the qualities reported in the PPN and the near-death literatures, participants would begin to see the remarkable similarity between the two. If they could grasp the possibility of memories and experiences reported during the near-death experience, they could start to consider the possibility of a similar type of experience coming into physical life.

The third study, by Dr. Jenny Wade, specifically addresses this comparison. Wade's "Physically Transcendent Awareness: A Comparison of the Phenomenology of Consciousness Before Birth and After Death" (1998) addresses the implications of evidence of memory (1) prior to brain development during the prenatal period, and (2) during near-death experiences in which the individuals' central nervous systems were not supporting life. In the case of the near-death experiences, only experiences reported that could be verified independently by a third-party were used.

Wade found the similarities between the two states striking in terms of attitudes towards life, self-boundaries, concept of other, and level of abstraction. Both were found to have concepts of others that were "fully mature, insightful, telepathic knowledge of other's mind, compassionate, records and processes information without emotional loading or neurotic projection" (p. 271). It is interesting that from the transcendent perspective, similar to

Wambach's findings, Wade reported an unpleasantness about coming into the body and saw the physical body as sometimes alien. After reviewing and comparing early prenatal life memories and near death experiences, Wade concluded:

> These two states have similar phenomenologies, suggesting that a physically transcendent source representing individual consciousness predates physical life at the moment of conception and survives after death, and that its maturity and functioning do not directly reflect the level of central nervous system functioning in the body. (p. 249)

In each of the three research examples, the continuity of self, sense of self, and sentient nature prior to conception during the prenatal and perinatal period is reported. In Wade's article, the similarity of the memories of these early experiences and those reported in her select group of near-death experiences lends support for the continuity of the sentient self prior to and beyond biological human life based on phenomenological subjective descriptions.

Transcendental and Human Sources of Awareness

Thus far, we have seen numerous examples of sentient expressions during early PPN experiences. The question is then how do we understand and resolve the apparent discrepancies in traditional early development and PPN perspectives. Why are these perspectives so divergent?

I believe the fundamental key to this question is found in our understanding of the two perspectives of awareness and experience reported in the PPN literature. Let us return to Wambach's finding that 89% of study participants reported two separate and simultaneous sources of awareness. As Wambach reported, each voice appeared to have its own unique qualities and perspective. She reported that the transcendent voice characteristically was devoid of emotion and characterized itself as a disembodied mind hovering around the fetus and mother, being in and out of the fetus. Here is an example Wambach shares of one person's description from this vantage point:

> When you asked about the fetus, I saw it and nurtured it and watched out for it, and also was in it all the way a few times, but not most of the time. I came in much more after birth than before birth. When you asked about the emotions of my mother, I was clearly aware of them. She was a little sad and upset because of Dad not giving her enough attention, and she was also deeply happy. (1979, p. 107)

Wambach also identified a fetal human body perspective that was characteristically more visceral and filled with strong emotions. Here is an example of the birth experience reports that describe both the human perspective, a viewpoint that typically includes a greater sense of sensory awareness, and the transcendental perspective of omni-knowing:

> In the birth canal I felt tight and very constricted and I was aware of darkness. As soon as I emerged I saw very bright lights and heard loud noises. As soon as I was born, I was aware of other people's feelings. I was surprised to find that my mother didn't want me. People were impersonal. I think to myself, "This is going to be a lonely trip." I think I must have rushed into this life. (p. 126)

What is significant in this case, is that this person has related realizations and forecasts for her future here as the newborn. Her last statement then reveals an adult assessment of the larger picture. Here is one more example from Wambach's group concerning the birth experience:

> The birth-canal experience was fear of being closed in and wanting to be free. After I was born I felt cold and difficulty in breathing. My spirit came in to stay at the time of birth. But I was aware of the feelings of others in the delivery room. They didn't think I'd live, and I wanted to tell them that I would. (p. 132)

Thus in this example, we see the human perception of sensations, the transcendental awareness of other's feelings and thoughts, the sentient intention of wanting to communicate with them, and a innate knowing that the outcome would be the baby would live.

Several authors in the PPN literature have focused directly on the notions and implications of the transcendental voice and sentient nature in terms of formulating new developmental theories. Wade's theory, articulated in *Changes of Mind: A Holonomic Theory of the Evolution of Consciousness (1996),* is one of the rare human developmental stage life-span theories that is viewed through the lens of the development of consciousness and that incorporates knowledge gained from the PPN research.

Based on extensive empirical research, she orients her model around an intricate exploration of the evolving relationship between the two sources of awareness—the transcendental source and the human brain-based source—over the course of the human life. In her model, Wade describes nine potential holonomic developmental stages of consciousness unfoldment over the life span (1996). Although Wade's in-depth articulation is beyond the scope of this discussion, I would like to include some of her concluding comments:

> Evidence from various disciplines supports a dual form of consciousness, where a physically transcendent source of awareness and a brain-based source of awareness coexist in ways that may not be directly causal or physically linked according to the conventional understanding of Western medicine. Within that framework, the brain-based source changes over life, as the area dominating awareness moves through evolutionary graded structures that represent increased neurological capacity and order. ... The data from the empirical sources cited throughout this book suggest a composite progression for the dominant source of consciousness that can be summarized in linear time as follows:
>
> A physically transcendent source representing individual consciousness (personhood, life essence) predates physical life at the moment of conception and survives it after death.
>
> The development of a biological body imposes some limitations on this source by binding it to the body. The transcendent source of consciousness may orient itself to the body as sheathing of energy that interpenetrates the body at some level.
>
> The physically transcendent source has its own form of awareness, whose maturity is not directly reflective of the level of central nervous system functioning in the body. Its awareness is rather detached and highly insightful, but its phenomenology is inherently the world of dualism. It is capable of transcending physical limitations to some extent and of operating along with the brain-based consciousness....
>
> As the brain's strength in generating its own energy field increases, subjective awareness of the transcendent source

decreases. This may be due to the interference or "noise" of brain wave patterns, and especially to the narrative dominance of the left hemisphere.

Over the course of development, the brain-based source of awareness progresses through evolutionary graded structures. Although neural firings occur in all parts of the brain, the momentary contour of the brain's energy field is dominated by well-worn patterns that are associated with different parts of the brain, reflective their influence on the interpretation of the aggregation of inputs. Progress follows MacLean's model and is additive. Over the lifetime, the experience of consciousness moves from the R-complex to the limbic system to the neocortex, and finally to cortical entrainment and increasingly slow, orderly, hyper synchronic bioelectrical activity. Consciousness changes dramatically as increasing neurological capacity becomes available.

Some people have a natural proclivity that permits them certain types of access to the transcendent source of consciousness during life, reflected by characteristic EEG patterns unlike those of the general population. Others can develop access through disciplined training. ... Accessing the transcendent source permits experiences unbound by Newtonian spatiotemporality, such as psi or "miraculous" abilities ("mind over matter").

Experience of non-Newtonian realities from that source is integrated into the brain bound consciousness. At higher stages of consciousness, progressive integration of the transcendent source in conjunction with an ego-transcending motivation changes the brain's EEGs, entraining both hemispheres and creating slower, more orderly and harmonic energy patterns. (Wade, 1996, p. 249-251)

In these concluding remarks, Wade portrays an intricate, evolving relationship between the transcendental source of awareness and the developing biological source of awareness. I am grateful to Wade for her pioneering this model and the notion of the evolution of these two perspectives as foundation. As I considered what I believed best holds the body of PPN findings, my own experience, and the experiences my clients portrayed, I also came to believe, it is the relationship between these two perspectives that gives us the best foundation for building the Integrated Model here. In that way, I build upon Wade's orientation and theory. Now let us take this piece along with the various materials discussed earlier to begin weaving our new tapestry.

The Integrated Self: A Holonomic Synergy of Transcendent and Human Perspectives

Although a wide range of expressions of awareness and experience are reported in the PPN clinical literature, they migrate into the two sources of awareness: the transcendental perspective and the biological human perspective. Wade referred to the biological human perspective as the human brain-based source. I recommend broadening that reference of the "human brain-based" source to the "biological human perspective" so as to include cellular and somatic memory reported prior to and in accordance with brain activity.

One of the greatest gifts of the PPN clinical findings is the exploration of these two perspectives, the characteristics of each, and the relationship between them. In most PPN experiences reported, the description includes an intimate intertwining of both the transcendental and human perspectives, as Wambach's example did.

Let's take the example of Dr. Farrant's description of his

experience journeying down the fallopian tube as a zygote during his regression session. Dr. Farrant related simultaneously being immersed in (1) the somatic experience of physical movement patterns of the zygote, (2) the transcendental state of oceanic bliss, and (3) the sentient experience of choice as he paused to consider whether or not he wanted to go through with this life. Furthermore, PPN clinical work with babies and young children shows us how to relate and support their whole being by supporting and encouraging the integration of these perspectives.

In order to deepen our examination of these two perspectives, I have summarized numerous distinct characteristics of each perspective reported in the PPN literature in Table II, many of which have already been discussed above. This table is a work in progress; yet seeing the connections between the various characteristics even in this nascent stage is very useful. Before speaking directly about the table, I want to clarify some terms and issues that shape the discussion.

Many different terms have been used to indicate a multidimensional nature that is inclusive of these two sources of awareness. In past publications, I have used the term *Authentic Self*. Now the term that seems to capture this concept more accurately is the *Integrated Self*. In essence, the Integrated Model of early development is based on the premise that in order to better understand our human self, we need to consider it in its holonomic relationship to the transcendental self. There is a synergy in which the whole is more than the parts and the whole organizes the parts. If we fragment the biological human self, we have already distorted our understanding and dissociated part of our truer nature. During human life, we appear to have a holonomic, holographic

83

spectrum of experiences that are a synergy of the biological and transcendental sources of awareness and origins.

As discussed earlier, I am working from the premise that we have a transcendental self that has a sentient nature prior to conception of the human body and therefore human self. I define *Self* here as a sentient state of consciousness in which there is a sense of I AM. I am utilizing a portion of Dossey's definition of consciousness: "The capacity to react to, attend to, and be aware of self and other. ... A state or quality of being with a capacity for sentience and subjectivity" (2003, p. A11). (For a fuller definition of this and other relevant terms, see Appendix Terms and Definitions.)

Once the physical process begins, the two perspectives form a holonomic, holographic, self-organizing, dynamic self-system, what I refer to as the Integrated Self. As in any dynamic system, the Integrated Self is characterized by an ever-evolving relationship between the two, each informing and changing with experience and interchange of the other. During incarnation, the description focuses on two sources of awareness or perspectives. Within each of these perspectives, the vast complexity of energy and information coalesce as the Integrated Self during the human lifetime. After death of the human body, it is the premise of this model that the transcendental self continues as a differentiated sentient I AM consciousness that has retained memory of the experiences in the physical realm, continues to experience and evolve, and has been found to have the ability to communicate with humans and affect our physical world (see the Appendix Bibliography for further reading in this arena). I acknowledge that for some readers the premise of a sentient self outside of human life—before or after—is very controversial and might be seen as highly speculative and not "proven."

My description and discussion of the transcendental Self and perspective is very general in this publication. In this book I refer to the implicit and explicit orders of existence. There is evidence to suggest that there are many planes or levels of nonphysical transcendental experience and existence that are each qualitatively different. In spiritual empiricism, these planes are more precisely explored and differentiated (various levels of experiences at the soul and spirit levels).

I also want to recognize the understanding in spiritual empiricism that speaks to a point in our evolution, where the I AM becomes more and more integrated into the collective I AM, into the ONE I AM (Wilber's *Eye of Spirit*, 2001, is one source to read further on this subject).

Also, it is important to be clear that our understanding of the transcendent perspective reported here comes from adult's, children's, and infants' retrospective reports, observations, portrayals of and re-connection (resonance) with these previous experiences during their pre-conception, prenatal, and perinatal experiences. This presents us with several important issues:

1. Our understanding of the transcendental perspective is *filtered* through the human body-brain-mind, through our human observing and measuring devices.

2. These reports then do not represent the fullness of the original experience, transcendent experience, or transcendental self, only the aspects that can be perceived, observed, and expressed through our human form at the time of the report. It appears that only a small portion

of our Integrated Self's original experience can actually be brought to conscious awareness and articulated or portrayed.

3. Even though we cannot bring these original experiences to full consciousness, the holographic recording and processing of the fuller experience is recorded, has impact, and is theoretically retrievable.

4. Memory of an original experience is always different from the original experience itself by its very nature as a dynamic feedback system that is very adaptable and changes with new information. However, this does not negate the potential accuracy or likeness of our memory or re-connection to the original event.

5. A complex yet important question arises: Does the sense of self in the memory come from the person's current orientation of self (whether an adult, child, or even infant) as he or she resonates with the earlier memory? Or is this a case of relating the sense of self that was present at the earlier age? I believe both are true and suggest giving consideration to this issue in the examples provided.

As we shift to a discussion of the material in Table II, the information reviewed in Chapter III helps to provide a framework of understanding. Table II is a culmination of PPN research, consciousness research, understandings from new physics, and my direct experiences, both personal and professional. As I tried to grapple with the complexity of it all, I found it very helpful to sit with each of the characteristics I have listed and consider my findings in terms of which perspective, transcendental or human, appeared to be involved.

I have included fourteen characteristics: domain, quality, vantage point, perspective, emotional tone, level of consciousness, sense of self/other, locus of control, awareness, perception and perspective, comprehension and stance, memory, communication, and Wilber's area of inquiry. For each of these characteristics, I found unique and distinct differences between the transcendental and human perspectives.

Although I pull them out separately here for our examination, I see them functioning in a fashion similar to the holographic process we discussed in the last section in which one pure beam of light is split into two beams of light. One beam of light experiences a three-dimensional object and reflects this information onto the photographic plate, the human perspective. The other beam remains as pure light and is reflected onto the plate, the transcendental perspective. As their information (perspectives) interact on the plate, they form interference patterns of encoded information that, when illuminated by a light source, provide the holographic image. Each perspective is necessary, and only in the synergy of their coming together is a reality created out of the chaos of all possibility. States of well-being and wholeness, I would suggest, involve the optimal flow and relationship between them.

Thus, in Table II I attempt to describe the qualities of each perspective, yet reality is a synergy of the two and represents more than the sum of the parts. Let's now look at these characteristics in more detail. I also encourage the reader to review the stories I shared earlier in the book in light of the information presented in Table II.

Table II

Prenatal and Perinatal Perspectives:
Reported Characteristics

Characteristic	Transcendental	Biological Human
Domain	Implicit, non-local, nontemporal, nonspatial, nonlinear	Explicit, local, temporal, spatial, linear, within time/space
Quality	Ethereal	Energetic, visceral
Vantage point	Outside human body	Inside human body
Perspective	Witness	Immersed in experience
Emotional tone	Devoid of strong feelings; love, caring, compassion portrayed	Strong emotions and responses
Level of consciousness	Super consciousness	Unconscious, developing subconscious-to-conscious
Sense of self/other	I AM consciousness; sense of transcendental self clearly differentiated from human body, human experience, physical environment and other humans; ever present continuous Self	Undifferentiated and fused with mother/ environment; own experience also; sequential development of ego-I human self
Locus of control	Proactive; capable of conscious intention, initiation, choice, action, orchestrating human self, yet allowing of the story to unfold, even if traumatic	Instinctual, reactive, responsive, adaptive
Awareness	Omni-transcendental awareness	Human awareness through biological human perception and senses processed through heart/brain/body

Perception and perspective	Capable of omni-extra-sensory perception and knowledge of: thoughts, emotions, intentions of others (especially parents), access to conscious, sub-conscious, unconscious, and intentions of others, environment, events with detail; functioning and awareness in both physical and nonphysical realms	Fused with human experience and environment; somatic, energetic, electromagnetic, fluids, cellular, tissue, chemical, hormonal, human body; primary knowing at somatic, energetic and physical levels
Comprehension and stance	Holonomic and holographic; primary knowing; ability to simultaneously comprehend the whole and every part, appreciating the larger picture as well as the smaller one; highly insightful, holds complexity, mature, loving, ethical, compassionate	Nonreflective, instinctual, adaptive, responsive; primary knowing at somatic and energetic levels
Memory	Non-local; not dependent on CNS functioning or physical body; holonomic and holographic; reflective-explicit possible with attention-intention-when observed	Local, instinctual, nonreflective, implicit, somatic, holonomic and holographic
Communication	Telepathic, mind-to-mind, intentional, not dependent on human physical form, yet uses it as a vehicle of communication as maturation supports	Through human per-ceptions, senses, and somatic expression: chemical, energetic, elec-tromagnetic, movement, gestural, voice (sounds, language), through reso-nance and states of being
Wilbur—area of inquiry	Spiritual and mental empiricism	Mental and sensory empiricism

As described in the table, the transcendental awareness appears to function in the non-local, implicit order of reality, and exists prior to incarnation. This vantage point expresses *I AM*, a mature sense of self, and clearly differentiates Self from the developing human body. This *I AM* perspective is consistent in its nature and its presence. I refer to it as the transcendental Self, or the primary non-local Self.

Regardless of maturation of the human brain or physical body, the transcendental Self, appears to have capacity of: functioning outside of time-space and three dimensional reality; primary knowing and gestalt holistic awareness—a holonomic, holographic ability to simultaneously comprehend the whole and relationships within the whole, while demonstrating insightfulness, ethical understanding, complexity, and maturity.

The transcendent voice is absent of strong emotions and portrays a witness perspective with tones of caring, compassion, and love that accompany the omni-wisdom characteristic of this perspective. Also characteristic of the transcendental level is the capacity for mutual and intentional mind-to-mind communication, omni-extrasensory perception and knowledge that include thoughts, emotions, and intentions of others. This suggests apparent assess to subconscious and unconscious levels of parents and other persons in the environment.

Referencing Mitchell's quantum holographic framework, there is evidence that suggests this transcendent awareness is operating prior to conception and is therefore *the primary awareness*, one that taps information prior to and after conception and demonstrates an omni-awareness that is far more expansive than the human cells and growing fetus can explain.

I would suggest therefore that this *perception* of non-local information is, as Mitchell suggests, our "first sense." In that way, perhaps our first sense of *implicit perception* is to our physical five senses as our mind is to our brain. This finding has extraordinary far-reaching implications for early development models and our ideas of how best to meet the baby's needs during life in the womb and infancy.

Now let us consider the contrasting human awareness characteristics. Whereas the transcendental Self's being, awareness and capacities appear consistent, ever present, and timeless, the human awareness begins with conception and evolves through a sequential developmental unfolding. The domain of the human self is within local time-space physical plane. Human level of reported awareness is oriented within the physical form and physical-emotional experience. During prenatal development, it is instinctual, non-reflective or implicit, somatic-emotional, adaptive, and at the core—relational. The human self appears to have a synergistic awareness that arises from it's own experience in relationship and a fused undifferentiated experience with the mother's and the environment: somatic, energetic, electromagnetic, fluid, cellular, tissue, chemical, hormonal, and sensory, and emotional awareness and responsiveness.

Communication is through energetic, electromagnetic, chemical, movement, gestures, and voice that evolve with development. The human self's experience is somatic, visceral, with intense emotions, and is intricately related and responsive to mother's experience, the health of the womb environment, the outer environment including other people, and the physical/emotional journey at birth. Although highly adaptive and responsive, there is also intentional, volitional, and conscious awareness, intention, and communication.

Once incarnation begins, these two distinct vantage points of the transcendental Self and human self give rise to a holonomic, holographic spectrum of awareness and experience, as an evolving nonlinear dynamic self-organizing system of being, what I have called the Integrated Self. Often traumatic experiences and imprinting are seen as a disruption or distortion of the natural flow between these levels of being and awareness.

Now let us continue our exploration of the significance of understanding these two perspectives. Traditional early development has focused primarily on the human level described above. Yet, with that narrowed focus, not only is the sentient transcendent Self not acknowledged or understood, but also, the implications of the synergy that comes with the capabilities of the transcendental Self and the needs of the human self in utero are not addressed. One of the most powerful understandings and frequently reported findings in the PPN clinical literature is the ability we have from pre-conception on to perceive information about our parents (and generations before) that appears holographic in nature, including all levels of the parent's being—conscious, subconscious, unconscious, explicit, and implicit patterns and memories.

The information may focus on one component, but includes physical, mental, emotional, and spiritual components. The information may be current, past, or sometimes future and appears to have non-local properties. (See Dossey's definition of non-local in the Appendix Terms and Definitions.) Because of our resonance with our mother and father through our DNA and our intimate ongoing relationship with mother while in the womb and as infants, we appear to have an incredible access to a wide spectrum of information about them. Most of the examples given earlier illustrate this ability.

Remember the story of Stevie who played the game portraying his conception with a diaphragm, yelling, "Ready or not here I come!" as he and his dad charged the fort? As his mother began to talk about when she discovered she was pregnant with him and tried to soften the expression of how she had felt, he interrupted her and blurted out "You were mad!" Some part of him knew the circumstances and knew her intense reaction to discovering he was here. One of the most consistent findings in the PPN literature is the knowledge we have of our parents' reaction to discovering we are here. This becomes a powerful element in our developing relationship, our view of self, and dramatically shapes our lives.

I want to share one more personal story related to my own PPN experience that illustrates the access to parental information and the ability to make life choices from the beginning of human life. One of my first regressions was of my conception during the second training module with William Emerson in 1990. I was still fairly new to PPN and did not have a lot of preconceived notions of what I would experience.

During the regression, I was stunned by information I "knew" about my mother's unresolved issues from childhood and unresolved pain. I later confirmed this with her. During the regression, I remembered having the sense as I came into relationship, with my parents and the conceptus back then, of getting a "gestalt download" of information, much of it not on an explicit level, yet having a sense of "intuitive knowing" about it. The piece about my mom's painful past became explicit, however. It felt as if it was a core part of our connection and relationship and purpose for being together. It also seemed to activate some "theme" that was to be a significant part of my life's journey. What happened next in the regression surprised me even more. I realized that at that time of the download and intuitive knowing, I had made a choice, a decision, and a commitment. I had felt a tremendous love and caring for her.

In that moment, I decided that I wanted to help her, to ease her pain. I would hold it with her. "I would carry her pain." In 1990, when I realized this, it had a profound ripple effect. I had been my mother's protector all my life, her source of "light" as she would say. I grew up feeling the pull to ease her pain.

After that regression, I was able to make a new choice and begin to differentiate constrictive versus expansive love and caring for her. Yet the experience still stunned me with the awareness of the elements of it all—the intuitive knowing of her life events and her inner emotional state, the sense of download of a tremendous amount of information, and the fact that I had made a life choice at that point. The implications were staggering.

As I continued my PPN training and reading, I found it a common phenomenon. In fact, I believe Emerson coined the term, "the fetal therapist syndrome," owing to the fact that so many people make adaptive choices during their experience in the womb—life stance choices that shaped their future. It appears that we are already making adaptive choices to meet the unmet needs of our mother or father and taking on self-identity roles in the family during this very formative time in the womb.

Here is an example of this phenomenon that comes from *Voices from the Womb* by Michael Gabriel (1992). This section contains both the words of the client, Katie, while remembering under hypnosis her experience in the womb, and the therapist's comments about her experience:

94

It's dark, with little or no energy. I'm cold, trying to generate warmth. I was so excited to come, to have the chance to love and be loved. Now I am trying to figure out what is wrong. This will be harder than I thought.

Katie spoke of her mother: "She is cold and clinical about having me; not excited and loving. She shows no feeling toward me." Nor was the mother better with her husband. Katie said:

She is not expressing herself with her husband. She is afraid of being vulnerable and blocks her feelings. When my father senses her love, what she does is she shuts down. She is disarming the person who loves her! She thinks she needs to keep strong, which to her means not feeling. All of her energy goes to maintaining herself and being in total control.

The marriage was already in trouble. Even so, Katie saw that her father was excited about his unborn child. She had a definite approach to the marital conflict: "I want to come out and convince my dad to stay." She took on the responsibility of keeping the family together.

How did Katie view her mother's lack of connection with her? Katie took the blame. She said:

It's very frustrating for me. I have an intense need for an intimate relationship with my mother, but I'm not getting it. I am not wanted or loved. I wonder what's wrong with me. There must be something wrong with me. [*This is in spite of the fact that Katie "knew" it was her mother's problem.*]

In the face of this, Katie was very courageous. She said:

The less I get from my mother, the more I try. Inside myself I feel confused and unwanted. Outwardly, I feel I need to do something. I take on a mission. My mission is to save their marriage, to keep my father there. It's real exciting—I will save her marriage. (1992, pp. 64-65)

Here is one more example of this important concept as described in *Cosmic Cradle*. Sage is sharing her inner knowing and the adaptive way of being in the family that she apparently set in motion prenatally:

My father and my mother's sister had a sexual affair during my mother's pregnancy with me. My mother denied the affair. She knew, but she did not want to consciously know. She felt terrified. ...

I told Mom that I was aware of dad's affair during my womb-time. She said, "Yes, you are right. They started their affair when you were in the womb, but I didn't not find about it until five years later."

Because I knew about the affair, I tried to babysit my father through it. As a child, I did things like sitting in between Dad and my aunt at church. During childhood, I felt angry towards my mother for being unconscious about it, but she contended with it as soon as she could. (p. 520)

These stories represent the type of adaptive choices we make very early during our experiences in the womb. The dynamics involved in this awareness of parents' inner feelings and dynamics between them with respect to the choices children make are very interesting.

What I find fascinating is the complexity here: on the one hand, we have access to an expansive scope of information about our parents and others and a sophisticated understanding of the dynamics involved often from the transcendental perspective; at the same time, as we come into the human domain with the information encoded in our DNA and the experience of being in the body and field of our parents, we appear to lose our more coherent sense of self and take on certain human beliefs and patterns. Through our fused state with mother, we resonant with certain states of being or patterns and imprint them as our own. In addition, we appear to make intentional assessments and choices that appear to be *adaptive* choices that will shape our growing beings from then on. We take on constricted beliefs, roles, and images of self. These become life patterns and appear to focus our attention and shape our lives.

A very common constricted belief we hear a lot in the PPN work is, for instance, "Something is wrong with me." Two common situations that give rise to this belief include (1) the discovery of a pregnancy in which the baby is unwanted, rejected, or a source of resentment or shame, and (2) the separation of baby and mother at birth. It is common in the early development community to consider the child vulnerable to the assumption that they did something wrong or are somehow at fault when something happens that is difficult to cope with, e.g., neglect or divorce. What we see in PPN clinical work is that we are vulnerable to these interpretations from the beginning of life.

Could it be that our need for love, connection, being seen, and welcomed is so strong from the beginning of life that we make these constrictive choices or beliefs to cope, that we would do anything to be connected and in a relationship? Cell Biologist Bruce Lipton (2001, 2005) tells us that our cells are directed by their perception of their environment from the beginning of life (www.brucelipton.com). If they perceived the environment as safe, they function towards growth. If their perception is it is not safe, they function towards survival.

Thus, from the human perspective, we are incredibly sensitive to our environment and dynamics; from a cellular level, or a psychic level, we are responding and adapting to our environment. When it is constricted or distorted, we adapt. In these interactions we develop beliefs about environment that shape our orientation towards protection or growth.

97

In our last example, Sage related a story in which she adapted to the psychological and relational dynamics of her parents. Another all too common theme in PPN work is the conflict experienced in the womb, at birth, and as an infant when life-sustaining needs are not met, resulting in a tremendous double-bind dynamic.

This next story focuses on the baby's experience in a chemically toxic womb and the ensuing broad spectrum of lasting impact. Often when there is chemical or emotional/mental toxicity at the moment when we implant in our mother's womb and come into connection with our life source, a deep conflict arises and a major adaptive strategy is put into motion to cope with the dilemma. When I teach this material to graduate students, I have them examine a life-long constricted belief and pattern they have had that potentially stems from their PPN period. One student who had done a lot of her own personal work with her PPN experience and issues, writes insightfully of her experience in the womb and the ensuing patterns:

> The belief that I have been looking at is my belief that "the world is not safe." The most blatant cause of this perception is the experience of being inside my mother's very toxic womb. She smoked between 1 and 1 1/2 packs of cigarettes per day. The sensation for me was of continually being singed by the nicotine. It was extremely painful and very debilitating. It caused me to breath shallowly in the womb and to squeeze my umbilical cord shut. I feel that I almost died several times during my gestation. I was malnourished because I couldn't allow myself to ingest large quantities of nutrients from my mother since everything was laced with nicotine. Her womb was therefore a danger zone for me. I could not control or stop her smoking and I never knew when the next attack would come. I was so weak at birth that I feel that I almost died.

These experiences have affected my entire posture of living. Below is an outline of some general ways in which I have been impacted by these early imprints:

1. I often relate to new experiences with fear, always evaluating the danger before anything else. This is of an obsessive proportion. I have spent my life in a fight or flight readiness for attack and my autonomic nervous system has been in a continual rev.

2. I have suffered from the condition known as "tactile defensiveness" and have spent most of my life holding a lot of tension in my body and not being able to be touched in certain key places.

3. My relationships have been fraught with a certain kind of anxiety and inability to let down into them. I have managed my relationships with extreme caution, unable to trust that they were safe and expending tremendous energy to make sure they stay non aggressive or antagonistic. Settling in with another person in an unguarded and vulnerable way has been very difficult for me.

4. My relationship to nourishment has been deeply confused and dysfunctional. I have not known what it means to really integrate nourishment into my body. I have had a love/ hate relationship with eating and food, which manifested in 12 years of bulimia and vomiting 5 times/day. I stopped vomiting 17 years ago and it has just been in the last four years that I have been feeling my authentic desires for nourishment and exploring what it means to respond to them.

5. I have had difficulty settling into, and being in my body. I have spent many years living outside of my body where there is no physical pain and exploring other realms of my consciousness. This has actually been very beneficial but now my experiences with consciousness must become grounded in my body.

I have been exploring these issues consciously and continually during the past six years and have made dramatic shifts. There are still some shifts that need to be made but overall I am feeling that I have finally arrived into my life and a sense that it is safe to be here.

This is a powerful portrayal of the lifelong effects of developing in a toxic womb. Notice that her first adaptive strategy in the womb is to try and control what is coming into her body. When this is not sufficient, she leaves. She disconnects from her human perspective and moves her attention into the transcendent awareness. The problem with this adaptive pattern is that it often leaves the person with a lifelong double-bind strategy. Often these people have a strong spiritual connection or psychic abilities and "like to hang out" there.

The difficulty occurs when they want to be in their body because they have to come back into contact with the trauma. When we are working with trauma from this period, what we see is an adaptive disruption of the connection between the two perspectives. Often a person experiences one of these perspectives without the awareness of the other.

In this student's case, her life pattern was to attend to experience in the transcendent perspective to cope with the tremendous suffering she experienced when grounded in her body. When her awareness is more grounded in her human perspective and body, the pattern is so powerful that she again, like the young baby, becomes immersed in it and loses the witness side of her experience and her ability to come into relationship with the pattern.

The following story from the human perspective also illustrates the powerful merged state we are in as we develop in our mother's womb, resonating deeply with mother's patterns. This is part of Dora's story under hypnosis of being inside her mother from *Voices from the Womb*:

> My mother has real doubts about life, wondering if it is worth being alive. She tremendously lacks self-worth. And yet she strongly wants to have this baby. She sends love to me but she can't love herself. I pick up on it. I don't differentiate between the love that's being sent and the self-hatred. The messages are intertwined. … Yeah, I'm taking it all in. That message, "I don't like myself," the tension, all the negativity is absorbed by me directly. … Her self-hatred is just one more thing I'm absorbing. …It permeates everything! I have this core feeling of not being okay. It's base level—the knowledge is almost irrefutable. It's from my earliest consciousness. I am not okay. (pp. 50-51)

This story powerfully illustrates it is more than talking to the baby or loving the baby, it is a state of self, a *state of being*, that the baby resonates with and imprints during pregnancy, birth, and infancy.

Thus far, we have focused on many of the characteristics of our transcendent and human perspectives. Let us now turn to our early capacity to communicate. The transcendent perspective's communication is telepathic, mind-to-mind. There are many examples of this in the PPN literature that display similar qualities and methods of communicating as the telepathic communication studied between adults in controlled settings.

In mind-to-mind communication, the mother or other receivers of the baby's communication can have that *first sense perception*, that intuitive knowing the baby is communicating. Sometimes this is received at an instinctual, non-reflective level and responded to at that level. Other times the communication is more explicit mind-to-mind communication in which the mother consciously senses the baby communicating with her. Communication often takes place during dream state, meditation, or daydreams. These mind-to-mind communications are often received by the mother (or receiver) in concordance with a spontaneous sense of emotional/physical states of the baby, a compelling sense to act or do something, and/or other more physical ways of communicating, such as kicking or changes in movements in utero.

I had a very sad story about this in my practice. A woman came to see me two months after losing her baby during her 37th week of pregnancy. She related that she had had a sense that something was not right, yet did not trust it. One day, she thought the baby was clearly communicating to her that she (the baby) needed help. That night, she felt the baby communicate, "I'm hanging on." Although she was up most of the night worrying about this, she hesitated to trust that that was truly her baby communicating to her and said, "How could I call the doctor and tell him my baby said she is in trouble?" She felt they would have thought she was "loony."

Sadly, during a previously scheduled ultrasound the next morning, the tragedy was revealed. The baby had her cord wrapped around her neck three times and had just died. From my point of view, this outcome may have been prevented if we understood and embraced the transcendent nature of our young babies and how natural telepathic communication with and from babies actually is. I am drawn to Somé's African village and their intentional attunement with the baby growing in the womb as they each invite and listen for the baby's communications.

Although the discussion of the two perspectives' characteristics here has focused mostly on illustrations from the period during pre-conception and prenatal life, earlier examples from Wambach's and Chamberlain's research portray similar multiplicity of capacities and sensitivities during birth and the newborn period.

Birth and bonding is a unique and critical developmental process in which the baby journeys from one reality to another—leaving the familiar and intimate womb world of mother, moving through her pelvis, and emerging to become a separate human being greeted by mother, father and others. From the PPN literature we see that during this metamorphic transition, babies experience and imprint in a heightened state of awareness, impressionability, and energetic permeability. What happens and how the baby perceives and responds to the myriad of moments during this developmental sequence in their journey of separation and reunion is etched into their psyche and their body at the deepest levels. From a PPN perspective, this journey serves as the inner blueprint for nearly every aspect of human life. If traversed well, it provides a positive foundation for core elements in the person's life. For example, birth and bonding is the spiritual journey in human form. It holds that archetypal journey of separation and reunion with Source and when supported and undisturbed, it can instill the innate confidence that "I can find my way home." It is also the map for what it means to move forward in life, to change, to move through challenges and "tight spots." It etches in whether we feel we are able to "meet the challenge," whether the journey of life feels like a lonely or loving one, and whether we look forward optimistically to future outcomes or not. How we are treated and valued for our gender, appearance, and the person we are, lays the foundation for self-worth and self-image.

How we are held, handled, spoken to, and listened to when we are born imprint and establish our subconscious beliefs of the stories our lives. Every aspect of the birth and bonding process and the newborn's experience from this multiplicity of perspectives becomes the foundation their body and psyche will rely on to guide them in life, often below the level of conscious awareness. Yes, birth and bonding is a very sacred journey in each human's life.

After their birth, babies continue to show us the abilities and characteristics of the two perspectives and the multiplicity of capacities. In my prenatal and perinatal work with babies I intentionally relate to the baby's Integrated Self, to the whole being with a transcendent Self that has that omni-awareness and perception and access to information at multiple levels, especially concerning their parents and others in direct contact. The acceptance of the fact that the baby has a sense of self, is capable of intentional local and non-local communication, is capable of understanding communication beyond what is previously thought, and who can learn, make choices and change his or her beliefs and patterns is essential to my practice.

I also hold the human self as one that is immersed in its experience, very merged with mother and its environment, exquisitely sensitive to its environment through first perceptions and senses, and has all the needs that we are familiar with in the early development community. In working with babies and their parents, we model this new way of *Being with Babies* (see my *Being with Babies* booklets published for parents to help with these new principles).

In my article *The Power of Belief: What Babies Are Teaching Us* (2002), which I have included as an Appendix, I suggest that by the time we are young babies, we have already established myriad

104

beliefs that shape our being at every level. These beliefs filter our perceptions and shape our sense of self, our relationships, our bodies, and every aspect of our development. I give four clinical examples of therapeutic work with babies that demonstrate their current resonance with earlier events and experiences that have created problematic patterns in their lives as infants. In those examples, I also discuss how we communicated and worked with the babies. Although I did not articulate the work quite in the same way back then, the examples illustrate our integrated approach to communicating and working with babies in which we are relating to the Integrated Self.

For most of us in the Western world, we do not know how to relate appropriately to the Integrated Self, the whole self. What does it mean to relate to a baby's Integrated Self? In some writings that speak to the transcendental nature of children, the children are characterized as "royalty." Certain qualities such as their heightened sensitivity, difficulties, and challenging behaviors are attributed to their special royal nature. I would suggest it is important to carefully consider where these characteristics originate. Often in working with babies and children these characteristics are actually trauma patterns originating in PPN experience which become part of the human self's imprinted constrictive life patterns. When we work with children utilizing a PPN-oriented assessment and intervention these characteristics resolve. Thus, I would caution assigning these characteristics to the transcendental nature of these children per se.

I remember one parent, upon hearing of these expansive capabilities, would call his son the little guru, or one mother who would ask her baby "Should we buy this house?" consulting her daughter as a psychic. I cautioned the parent that although the baby did have transcendental awareness and capacities, not to put too much responsibility and expectations to "read" situations on their baby's consciousness. I gently guide parents to appreciate both natures in balance. They are human babies, sensitive, with a need to be nurtured, loved, nourished, and attuned to. At the heart of our awareness of babies' transcendent capacities is the understanding that we can relate to babies in a much richer way when we are relating to their Integrated Self.

Chapter V

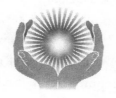

Integration

The ground upon which we build the Integrated Model of early development is the holonomic, holographic understanding that our physical human self is a part of, an expression of, our more expansive, inclusive, and primary transcendent Self. As we come into embodiment, our transcendent and human perspectives are in a holonomic, holographic relationship and become a self-organizing system I call the Integrated Self. The relationship is dynamic, creative, adaptive, yet always in the pursuit of greater connection, complexity, and wholeness.

During the modern era, an artificial split between these two perspectives developed and was reinforced generation after generation, creating morphogenetic fields of ways of being and believing, and narrowing perceptions of reality. Our knowing of this transcendent nature from the beginning of life and the understanding of how to attune and receive consciousnesses at this level diminished or was denied. The Newtonian models of physics and resulting models for medicine, psychology, and early development undermined connectedness and intuitive knowing, as the observable physical world became primary. As a result of this process, something most dear was forgotten.

Wilber suggests the challenge of our postmodern era is integration—the integration of science and authentic spirituality. Wilber's integral model gives us a framework to hold all three unique arenas of inquiry: spiritual, mental, and sensory empiricism. Within Wilbur's integral approach, we can honor the interiors of I and WE and the exteriors of IT in our inquiries.

Current understandings of the universe and human existence appear to be coming full circle, returning to the understanding that our physical reality is but one aspect of the greater quantum holographic universe and a mysterious All-That-Is from which we truly cannot be separated. We have come to understand that we perceive and utilize information not only in our local physical dimension, but also from the non-local implicit dimensions as well.

Science now shows us what mystics and shamans have practiced for centuries—that by bringing our attention and intention into focus, we have impact on our world and others regardless of time and space. With this and the thirst for re-connection with soul and spirit that we are witnessing, our morphogenetic fields are changing and the reconnection is gaining momentum.

Our current early development models are reflecting this movement towards integration and connection with the appreciation that our development is essentially dyadic in nature and that our early experiences create the architectural blueprint for life. The need to connect, yet follow our own rhythms and self in healthy attachment and self-regulatory patterns, speaks to the importance of our ability as parents and caretakers to attune and be in our most coherent self as we care for our young ones.

Much of the perspective of current infant development thinking has come from physical inquiry, behavioral and sensory empiricism, and observation and analysis. It remains rooted in the worldview that biology is primary and that the capacity for sentience is dependent on brain development. Although childhood spirituality and spiritual intelligence is gaining more attention (Hart, 2003), there is still virtually no mention of our primary consciousness, soul, spirit, or our transcendent nature in current mainstream infant development literature and education.

Prenatal and perinatal psychology has brought a tremendous renewal to the exploration of our understanding of human experience from an integrated lens that honors our multidimensional nature. In this exploration, we have also discovered the unfortunate-to-tragic repercussions that result from the separation of our human perspective from our transcendent perspective in the ways we have come to view babies, birth, and our ways of being with babies that deny their capacity, sentience, and accompanying needs during their incredibly impressionable early period.

The stories in this publication represent myriad human lives that, in their wake, have implications that call us to re-integrate, to remember, and to create new models and approaches that go beyond either the extraordinary advancements in science or the ancient wisdom of the Great Chain of Being. We now have an opportunity to create the best of all perspectives by bringing these concepts into integrated approaches.

Integrating Traditional Western
Early Development into the Integrated Model

As I return to my own journey of exploration of early development and the dissonance I have felt between the lens of early development and that of prenatal and perinatal psychology and what babies and children have taught me, I find that the integrated holonomic, holographic framework holds the best of each tradition. Each becomes more than it was separately when held within the greater whole of the Integrated Self. The exploration of the two perspectives of awareness in the prenatal and perinatal literature is tremendously clarifying. Now as I consider the perspective of current early development models within this holonomic, holographic Integrated Model, they come into focus in a new way.

For example, looking at the notion that we are totally fused with mother and the environment in utero and during early infancy and that we slowly gain a sense of self still feels true. The "ah-ha" moment for me was when I re-conceptualized that this is true for the human self. Development of object permanence over the infancy period exists as a developmental phenomenon for the human self.

Early development understanding in western cultures has focused on the human self, the biological self. From that lens, yes, these models are true in their domain and help us understand the process of learning to be human—in a human body, in a human family, in a physical, three-dimensional world! It also makes sense that as transcendent, sentient consciousness beings who exist beyond our time/space physical world, we need to learn be oriented to and taught how to function in the human body, in human relationships, and in the physical world. We also need to learn how to be human, to think, to feel, be in relationship and how to deal with the range of human emotions and responses. We begin this process merged with our parents, orienting to being human in our specific circumstances through our intimate connection to their experience while slowly developing our own ego-self, separate from our parents and our environment over time.

Thus, I believe we have these two distinct, yet intricately woven levels of awareness, and that much of what traditional western early models have focused on is the examination of human self-development. Now as we bring those human self-oriented findings into our integrated holonomic model, much of them hold their truth, yet there is now a greater truth in which they are held—that we are more than our biological self, that our sentient consciousness is primary, that our transcendent Self is present before and as we come into embodiment; AND, that we can come into more direct rapport and relationship with the sentient consciousness and meet them more fully.

When we broaden the lens to include both the transcendental Self and human self, our models of early development and how to best welcome consciousness reconstellate into a model that has greater complexity, coherency, integrity, self-organization, and reflects the truer dynamic of the holonomic, holographic nature of the relationship. That is my belief. That is my vision.

In our current understanding of brain development, we know the reptilian brain is the most active portion of the brain during early infancy. We also see that when the next higher level of brain functioning, the limbic brain, becomes more dominant in its activity and comes into relationship with the reptilian brain, it *reconstellates the functioning of the lower brain.* This incremental pattern

111

of re-constellation occurs as each level of the brain emerges as a focus of growth and activity. The importance of this holonomic view of integration of the four brains is one of the most significant findings in the early development community today.

When I sit with what babies and children have been teaching me, what holds the integrity of my direct experience with them in their healing processes is this holonomic principle. I believe the same holonomic principle holds true when we bring the biological human self into our Integrated Model, that it is reconstellated by the more encompassing and inclusive transcendent Self.

When we reconstellate our lens and our ways of supporting and being with babies that incorporate their (and our) more expanded and primary nature, their (and our) transcendent nature in relationship with their human nature, it reconstellates how the human self develops and functions.

This book has focused upon the fundamental premises needed to build our understanding of the multidimensional Integrated Self and the Integrated Model of early development. Upon this foundation, key aspects and issues need to be addressed and further explored. I introduce four key issues here: Early experience and the formation of the adaptive unconscious, need theory, the holographic spectrum of communication and learning, and implications for the model imperative principle.

Early Experience and the Formation of the Adaptive Unconscious

We develop in relationship to our environment. Whether it is a cell's perceptions of and responses to the environment (Lipton, 2005) or our primary intuitive perception of our parent's subconscious intentions, thoughts and feelings, our responses and choices shape our stance and living of life from then on.

Many of the adaptations appear to be constrictive ones to cope with unmet needs, unhealthy or toxic emotional and physical environments, unresolved parental issues, and traumatic events and interventions during the prenatal, birth and neonatal periods. We resonate with states of being of our mother and environment and can imprint them *as our own* patterns. (For a fascinating example of this, read the clinical story of Leslie in the Appendix *The Power of Belief*.)

More specifically, our spectrum of early experience and our adaptive responses to it form the foundational labyrinth-like structures of our subconscious, autonomic functioning—what some refer to as the adaptive unconscious (Wilson, 2002). Wilson defines the unconscious as the "mental processes that are inaccessible to consciousness but that influence judgments, feelings, or behavior" (2002, p. 23). He reports research indicating that our senses alone take in over 11,000,000 bits of information at any given moment, yet we can only consciously process 40 bits of information during each moment!

According to Wilson, the adaptive unconscious scans the vast amounts of information for patterns, organizes, interprets, evaluates, and prioritizes the information, and is capable of complex learning in the process—all at an unconscious level. A very complex set of operations not only directs what sliver of experience will be attended to at a conscious level, but what meaning and interpretation accompanies it. Wilson suggests that our adaptive unconscious develops "chronic ways of interpreting information from our environment" and that "highly energized" information appears to make it more "accessible" (p. 37).

This information gives us a deeper appreciation of the amazing power our subconscious and autonomic programming has in shaping our lives! When and how are these elaborate set of operations established? What determines the sliver of reality that we will be conscious of in any given moment?

I believe what Wilson refers to as highly energized chronic patterns are primarily formed during our earliest experiences. These findings reinforce the enormous importance our earliest experiences have in establishing life-enhancing and positive implicit memories and patterns. For example, for optimal development, having the experience and implicit memories of feeling wanted and welcomed, set in motion life-enhancing subconscious beliefs, meaning, and significance that effect the person's expectations and interpretations as they encounter new relationships and situations from that point forward.

The Integrated Self and Needs Theory

To support wholeness from the beginning of life and meet the needs of the Integrated Self during prenatal life and birth and bonding, we are also called to reconstellate our developmental needs theory. Developmental need theories in the 20th century traditionally began with the needs of the child or infant and did not address needs during prenatal life or the perinatal period. The theories were based upon the view of the human being as a strictly biologically based entity.

Our 21st century need theories address the needs of the Integrated Self from the beginning of life and appreciate that how we meet the baby's needs during the prenatal and perinatal period lay the foundation for postnatal development. As a holonomic, holographic being, the whole being is more than the sum of the parts, the whole organizes the parts, and the higher level of the transcendental Self holds a higher level of organization, complexity, and function than the human physical level. Thus, meeting the needs of this multidimensional being entails supporting the integration, the communication, and the connection between transcendental Self and human self. This begins with our holding the vision of babies' wholeness and the knowing that their human self is an aspect of their ever present transcendental Self.

As the transcendent Self, I believe we have an innate affinity for the spiritual aesthetics of love, joy, truth, beauty, freedom, clarity, balance and symmetry, light, compassion, kindness, and ethical justice. Our transcendental and human perspectives connect and flow most fully—and we thrive most fully—when our environment resonates with these.

This book began with the quote, "They don't know I am a person. I know I am." As I discussed earlier, when I reviewed what we have learned from the baby's perspective, this was the most fundamental message, and in essence points to our core, innate need to be seen as a person and to feel that we matter.

Within this understanding, many of the needs we have considered essential for healthy development during infancy and childhood we now see are needs from the very beginning of human life. PPN findings have consistently revealed that we thrive when we are welcomed, wanted, loved, and valued and related to as a person.

One of the most profound themes in spirituality and in the human journey is the journey of union–separation–reunion. As we separate from our spiritual world and come into physical life, the quality of how we are met, the quality of our first connections and relationships, and our experience in this physical domain are the foundations for our sense of safety, self-worth, belonging, and our capacity for empathy and positive relationships.

We thrive when we are engaged in relationships that are responsive, caring, and attuned with our needs and experience; when our parents are thriving and enjoying their lives and are whole enough to allow us to become who we innately are rather than to meet *their* needs. When our parents and others are in states of happiness, joy, well-being, love, appreciation, and health, we thrive. On the other hand, we move into constriction and survival adaption—developing our coping strategies—when we experience physical or emotional toxicity, rejection, conflict, domination, objectification, exclusion, fear, shame, violence, deceit, depression, or trauma, and feel alienated and alone.

Although formulating more precise needs theory is beyond our focus here, bringing attention to these core elements already begins to deepen our appreciation of needs and how we can best support the wholeness of babies as sentient beings and sensitive human beings.

Integrated Being and Knowing: Perceptions and Senses

In Chapter IV we began building our model with the two primary levels of experience: transcendent (non-local) and human (physical). To further clarify the spectrum of experience, I want to introduce another element of specificity here and speak to the energetic level of our being. From conception on, while in the womb, during birth and bonding, and during infancy, we perceive, function, communicate, learn, and have memory on the non-local consciousness, energetic, and physical levels. The transcendental level is primary, functions non-locally, and occurs instantaneously. The physical level in Table II includes both physical and energetic components.

The energetic view of reality and human life is receiving a great deal of attention during this century's first decade. Energy psychology and energy medicine focus on the human energy system that includes the enveloping biofield, chakra centers, and the meridian pathways. Together these create the human vibrational matrix. In research on information sharing and human experience, the energetic level has been found to transfer information more quickly than occurs at the physical level and is considered the bridge between the non-local and physical levels (Hunt, 1995). Although much of this discussion is beyond our focus here, let us add one additional element: heart intelligence and the implications for the Integral Model and early development.

The field of neurocardiology and the extensive research by the Institute of HeartMath reveal that the heart is not only a pump for our circulatory system, but also is a "highly complex system with its own functional "brain"... a sophisticated center for receiving and processing information" that learns, remembers, and makes functional decisions independent of the brain's cerebral cortex (McCraty, Bradley, & Tomasino, p 15). Brain rhythms have been found to naturally synchronize to the heart's rhythmic activity.

In ground breaking experiments, researchers at the Institute of HeartMath have demonstrated that both the brain and the heart's sensory neuronal system receive and respond to information about an event *before* the event actually happens (McCraty, Trevor, and Tomasino, 2005; McCraty, Atkinson, and Bradley,

2004). *In their experiments, the brain and the heart responded to randomized events seconds prior to the events even being chosen by the computer.* This suggests that the brain and heart had access to non-local information and were already responding to it before it moved from a potential wave quantum state into being an actual physical event within time-space. *Remarkably, the heart was found to respond before the brain did.* Thus the heart was shown to be the more primary responder to the non-local information. The researchers suggest that the heart's electromagnetic field, the strongest EMF in the body, may be "linked to a more subtle energetic field that contains information on objects and events remote in space or ahead in time" in what they refer to, as Edgar Mitchell does, "intuitive perception" (McCraty, Trevor, and Tomasino, 2004, p. 17).

Now let's take this information and consider perception and senses in light of our holonomic, holographic Integrated Model. I agree with Mitchell's suggestion that intuitive perception, or what some call primary knowing, is our primary "first sense." If we apply our holonomic model, intuitive perception is the perception of information at the quantum level, involving the highest levels of integration, self-organization, and complexity of the holonomic Great Chain of Being. Thus, when we are accessing and in alignment with it, we are functioning at those higher levels. We are tapping the domain of our transcendental awareness.

This is such a fascinating territory to explore. PPN memories clearly indicate we access and function at this level of omni-knowing and evaluation. Yet, could this non-local primary level of knowing relate to what many have called *innate intelligence?*

Lipton (2005) discovered that cells "know" whether the environment is safe or not. Applied kinesiology uses the principle that testing the strength or weakness of a person's muscle can be done in order to discovery if something is true or not. The system would test strong if the statement being tested is true, or weak if it is false. The strong-weak test is also used to assess if something enhances the person's well-being or diminishes it. These examples could be said then to be primary knowing at various levels of being. Babies and children often demonstrate their primary knowing when accessing PPN experiences, such as in the examples I gave of Beau and Ian. We are familiar with the primary knowing of our emotions, such as love. How do we know, we are asked? "We just know," is a characteristic response of a primary knowing.

One of the principles I first wrote about in *Being with Babies*, and is a principle I incorporate into every aspect of my work and teaching, is that genuine authentic truth helps us orient in our being in our Integrated Self. I have experienced this hundreds of times in my practice. When we create an atmosphere of caring, compassion, and sensitivity, and we recognize, acknowledge and share something that occurred or is occurring, it can be a profoundly healing moment. During the 20th century, when the predominant notion of babies excluded the possibility of meaningful memory, feelings, and responses to early PPN events or dynamics, most difficult or traumatic things were never discussed or acknowledged at the time or even later in life. When the truth is found and dealt with, such as occurs in PPN oriented therapy, the healing begins.

I would suggest that our innate intelligence is primary knowing informing every level of being and that it originates within the quantum implicit order. Thus when a truth is acknowledged, it creates an alignment of primary knowing between our transcendental Self and human self and a new, higher order of self-organization is possible.

119

At the physical level of awareness, awareness is traditionally thought of in terms of our five senses. A sixth sense, that is more fundamental, appears to be our perception and ability to orient in time-space. I would suggest that in between the quantum and the ability to orient in time and space and in our physical senses is our ability to perceive energetically or vibrationally. This includes the perception of subtle energy fields and electromagnetic fields, such as the heart's electromagnetic field. See Figure I below.

In the Integrated Model, this full range of perception and sensory awareness is seen to function synergistically at all levels of information sharing and communication: quantum, energetic, and physical. The more consciously we can attune to this full range of experiencing and knowing, we deepen our communication and attunement with babies' integrated nature and our own as well.

Figure I
Holonomic Levels of Awareness and Perception

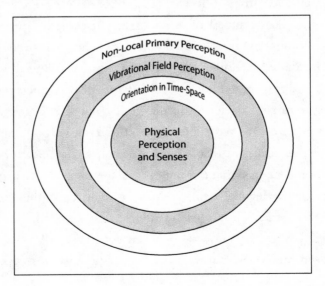

HeartMath research also adds to our understanding of states of being, attunement and our interpersonal communication process. Not only is does the heart function as a "brain," the heart also provides the body's most powerful rhythmic electromagnetic field (EMF), projecting its field out several feet from the body. Coherent heart states, as measured by beat-to-beat variability, are associated with positive states of being; love and appreciation promote greater systemic coherence. States of less coherence, such as frustration and anger, are associated with a disordered incoherence. The heart is seen to act as a carrier wave for information that provides a global synchronizing signal for the entire body intrapersonally.

They have also found that the heart's electromagnetic field transmits information between people up to five feet away and that the heart's nervous system actually acts as an "antenna" which is tuned to and responds to the electromagnetic fields of others.

There are many physiological and psychological implications of these findings. It could be suggested that the mother's state of being and her corresponding heart coherence acts as a carrier for her growing baby prenatally and postnatally. It is interesting to note that our heart begins beating at four weeks in utero. For nine months, we are patterning our heart patterns and states of being with our mother's. We are imprinting her carrier waves and our responses to them. As in their experiment in which the heart sensed the quantum information before the brain registered it and appeared to be acting at a more primary level of communication, during prenatal development, the heart is sensing and learning for months before the brain fully comes on line during the third trimester. Heart intelligence, heart perception, and primary knowing appear once again to be the more foundational bridge between our transcendent Self and our human self.

I believe the heart intelligence research is central to our deeper understanding of the holonomic, holographic Integrated Self and how to best support optimal wholeness from the beginning of life. Although it is beyond the scope of this text to develop this further, the Institute of HeartMath and the authors of the article cited above have graciously allowed me to include a succinct introductory article on their findings as the Appendix *The Resonant Heart*.

The Model Imperative Principle

The model imperative principle is a prominent one today in the early development literature. The mother's (caregiver's) state of being is seen to be the model, which the baby's brain and system comes into a dynamic relationship with and utilizes to build their own. The adult holds the integrity of the adult functioning brain, autonomic nervous system, and states of being for the baby to organize and regulate with.

I would extend this principle to say that adults' ability to be congruent, coherent, and to live from their Integrated Self—their ability to hold the integrity of this higher level of complexity and order in their state of being—provides a higher level of potential complexity, coherence, and integration for the baby's system to resonate with and build their Integrated Self. The heart intelligence literature also substantiates this broader view of coherence modeling by the adult for the baby (www.heartmath.org). For further reading on parenting with a focus on the primary importance of *state of being*, I recommend *Magical Parent, Magical Child: The Optimum Learning Relationship* by Joseph Chilton Pearce and Michael Mendizza.

The other important aspect of the model imperative principle comes from my direct experience with babies and children, along with related reports by my colleagues. When I hold the vision of babies from pre-conception on as multidimensional beings, having the integrity of transcendent and human perspectives, processes, abilities, and capacities, I come into resonance with more of who they are. I am expanding my awareness to come into relationship with their expanded spectrum of awareness and being. I am utilizing not only a greater awareness, but I am actively interacting with them at multiple levels—physical, energetic, and non-local. In that way, I experience and interact, and they show me more of who they are! That greater spectrum of being and awareness is what I believed I witnessed and felt within me as I watched the video of the baby with William Emerson so many years ago.

The Integrated Self:
New Horizons

What is possible when babies and children are related to, held, and understood in these integrative ways? We are just at the beginning of finding out. What we have considered the "norms" of early development have been based on babies who all too often have undiagnosed stress-trauma-shock patterns from their PPN experiences and unmet needs. Our narrowed view of babies have shut down so many avenues of their being met and encouraged, we really do not know what the new norms would be if we supported the Integrated Self. The expression, "use it or lose it" that has become popular in the new early developmental brain research seems applicable here. What potentials are lost or lie dormant waiting to be awoken?

In the last twenty five years, we have witnessed a surge of interest in spirituality and cultivation of our deeper relationship with Self and Source, as well as a welling drive to reawaken slumbering capacities of primary knowing, intuitive perception, and intentional healing, to name a few. Myriad programs and methods have been designed to develop more conscious dominion of these spectrum of experiences and capabilities during adulthood. Could it be that if we meet and nurture the Integrated Self more fully at the beginning of life, that we retain a much more conscious and fluid connection between our transcendental and human perspective? I believe so.

From my experience and that of my colleagues, it is safe to say that when we welcome consciousness, understand and meet prenates and babies as *sentient beings-sensitive human beings*, and live *Being with Babies* principles in ways that support their wholeness and rapport between their transcendental Self and human self, we see greater coherence, regulation, aliveness, resilience, connectedness, presence, mutuality, joy, open-heartedness, positive self-regard, enhanced abilities and creativity, intuitive knowing, and greater health.

From my experience with babies and children and their parents, profound changes can take place when we relate directly to the Integrated Self. In early development intervention models, most interventions are parent-oriented, with babies being "talked about" or "done to." When we come from an understanding of the Integrated Self, one of the simplest, yet most powerful shifts takes place—we include babies directly. In that shift another level of experience, healing, and imprinting life patterns emerges. When we consciously meet the Integrated Self, we enter a dance that includes the physical, but that becomes more—an exquisite physical, emotional, mental, and spiritual orchestral piece—a dance that not only attunes to the physical, but strikes the harmonics of the energetic and non-local notes as well. That synergy in and of itself offers greater possibilities and actualities. (This principle is highlighted in *Being with Babies, II.*)

Beatrice Beebe (1998), in the *Infant Mental Health Journal*, wrote of *the implicit relationship knowing* procedural mode. She writes of the special moment of meeting in which the two come into resonance together. One of the aspects of that resonance is the implicit relationship awareness that senses, "I know that you know that I know…" (p. 338). I find that this happens when I relate to babies this way. They know that I know they know and magic happens! Now I have come to believe this is what I saw in that baby's eyes 21 years ago at William Emerson's presentation of working with babies that changed me! Emerson and the baby had entered the "I know that you know that I know" in their conscious expanded *Integrated Selves.* And what I saw was gratitude for being seen at that level of being in that unique mutuality.

Why doesn't mainstream society understand or perceive this? This question brings me back to where I began, looking at the power of our beliefs. Remember our young doctor who believed the man had warts and successfully cured his warts, only to be told that wasn't possible by his attending physician? In that moment, he lost something, and no matter how often he went through the exact procedure again, no other patient was cured.

Over generations we were taught not to conceive or perceive our transcendental nature. We fell out of phase, out of resonance with this knowledge, and the ensuing empirical/scientific orientation of our early development research inhibited a return to this aspect of our reality. With our own prenatal and birth imprinting in a culture and world that has lost touch with this knowledge, most of us have lost our fuller connection with our truer nature as multidimensional beings as we fused with the DNA and parents who had lost their connection—and so the story goes.

My hope is that we are beginning to remember and reawaken more of who we are and can then welcome consciousness in a way that better supports babies' whole being from the beginning of life.

I plan to continue this discussion, articulating more aspects of the Integrated Model in greater detail and addressing a range of fundamental developmental topics pertaining to the Integrated Self, such as incorporating PPN and Integrated Self principles into assessment and interventions with babies, children and adults.

For now, let me say, when I look at the process of coming into human life, it is such a beautiful "plan." Here is a story I imagine about it all. Our consciousness, our transcendent Self, originates in the non-local spiritual dimensions that are outside our time/space dimensions in a much more expanded form. We choose to come into human form to experience Self through the experience of the Integrated Self—that intertwining of perspectives through human life. In order to be human in a physical world, we have to grow a body and learn to use our body and our physical senses. We have to learn how three-dimensional reality works, how to function where there is a past-present-future, where objects tend to stay and hold their form—object permanence. We have to learn how emotional-mental relationships work and we need to learn these not just generically; we need to learn them very specifically in order to live in our family, community, historical moment, and culture.

A beautiful plan. We are made of man and woman. We receive an incredible download of knowledge and information in our DNA. We attach ourselves and live in our mother's womb, resonating, listening, learning, and responding. By the time we are born, our relationships and views are already shaped, preparing us for our life and setting in motion life focuses and challenges.

Birth, that oh-so-physical journey, etches our blueprint of what movement from the known into the unknown will mean. And as we are born and connect with our mother and self-attach at her breast, we learn that even when we separated from our source, we innately know how to "find our way home and reconnect."

It truly is a beautiful plan.

I want to share one of Somé's descriptions of her tribe's rituals of welcome:

> The Dagara believe that what happens to us at birth and while in the womb actually molds the rest of our lives....
>
> Just like the preparation for pregnancy, the welcoming of the newborn is crucial. Indeed, in the Dagara tribe the first cry of the baby is critical. It is not seen as a simple cry, but as a coded message that is delivered upon arrival. In the village, children of up to five years of age are placed in the room next to the birthing room to answer the baby's first cry. They respond by crying back the way the baby cried, seen as answering the call and letting the newborn know it has arrived at the right place....
>
> Children are close in age to newborns and remember their connection to the spirit world. Therefore, it makes sense that they would be the ones to welcome the newborn. The Dagara people believe that our wounds of abandonment start at this early state of life, and so welcoming of the newborn by children and the

entire village at this early time in life is critical to the newborn's development.

... If the first cries of the newborn are not responded to, the psyche interprets this to mean that no one is there for it. Therefore, an unanswered cry leads to a deep wounding of the soul and later will translate at the community level as anger or violence in some form. (pp. 58-59)

One of the mentors who I trained with is Dr. Peter Levine who originated Somatic Experiencing™, a healing modality for working with trauma that is integrative. In *Waking the Tiger (1997),* he writes of the healing vortex and the trauma vortex. A helpful image is an infinity sign on its side with each loop as one of the vortex. If one becomes entangled in one or the other, the trauma vortex or the healing vortex, one is out of balance. Balance is found in the coherent flow between and the relationship at the center, in the relationship between these two vortices. It reminds me of the student's description of her traumatic beginnings inside her mother's toxic womb. She could get stuck in the trauma of being in her human experience that was built on a house of trauma-based imprints, or she could leave that focus and explore the transcendent experiences. It appeared to be an either or situation.

In trauma, we lose our center, the connection of our human self AND transcendental self. We lose the coherent flow of energy BETWEEN our aspects of our Integrated Self. When we lose the knowing of our transcendental nature, we lose the connection with our witness perspective and our ability to come into relationship *with* as well as be in the human experience. In healing trauma, we hold the witness perspective for and with the person if they move towards being immersed in their trauma experience. In being with

128

babies and holding their Integrated Self, we hold their witness transcendental self with them directly. This is a fundamental aspect of healing and imprinting more integrated ways of being.

Children who have been related to in this way in PPN-oriented interventions appear to have a greater capacity to consciously hold more of the fluid connection between their human and transcendental perspectives than commonly seen. They also appear to retain a more conscious access to the witness perspective as a way of being throughout their developmental stages. The implications of this are so significant that further discussion about this aspect is planned in further writings.

I recently came upon an advertisement for an upcoming workshop with Peter Levine. The title of his talk was "From Trauma to Awakening and Flow: Clinical Implications of Trauma and Spirituality." The description fits so beautifully that I include it here:

> The treatment of trauma is fraught with pitfalls and "tight corners." Generally overlooked, however, is a vital resource—the intrinsic relationship between trauma and spirituality. This intimate association suggests therapeutic avenues that support authentic transformation of traumatic experience. Once contacted, the "flame of the deep self" can re-ignite. In this way the vast energies locked in trauma can be liberated, acceded and integrated. When appropriately guided, our intrinsic wholeness is awakened offering profound healing resources for even the deepest trauma. This transformative process, of moving from trauma to awakening, offers the tangible possibility of becoming more whole than before a devastating event. (www.nicabm.com)

Towards the end of the 20th century, prenatal and perinatal psychology's clinical research brought tremendous renewal to the exploration of our understanding of human experience from an integrated lens that honors our multidimensional nature echoing the ancient wisdoms held in many indigenous cultures. Sadly, we have been witnessing the unfortunate-to-tragic repercussions of the modern western world's loss of that knowing.

As we begin the 21st century, we have the opportunity to better meet and support the Integrated Self and to set in motion a holographic blueprint of greater wholeness and rapport with Self from the beginning of life. Consider if this were to become the norm—if our attunement and our ability to perceive, communicate and have dominion more consciously at all three levels: physical, energetic, and quantum, became part of our natural daily ways of being—what would be possible then? This exploration takes us into new western frontiers, beyond what indigenous cultures have known. We certainly can gather the riches from indigenous cultures, yet we need to find our own paths in the 21st century's information age terrain.

I believe one of our first steps is to clear the land of outdated western beliefs and premises that stand in the way of cultivating the fuller vision of who we are. Nurturing the possible, supporting the integrity and wholeness of the Integrated Self from the beginning of life, opens the door to help each new being create a foundational holographic blueprint that supports their fullest creative life force and wholeness. I hope you will join me in welcoming consciousness. The territory is ripe for further exploration.

We began with Emily's statement, "They don't think I'm a person. I *know* I am." In my being with babies, I want them to know that I know that they know that they are sentient, conscious, aware beings.

In closing, I believe we are never too young or old for the need for the nurturing of being seen, heard, touched, valued, and included. When we honor the wholeness of our baby's spirit as their body is conceived and as they are nurtured in the womb and birthed; when we treat them with love and respect and include them as whole, sentient beings that are learning intensely about life and communicating with us from the beginning; and when we appreciate their conception, womb life, and birth as their unique sacred journey into human life, we can compensate when everything doesn't go well, when "life happens." When we nurture the wholeness, the goodness, truth, and beauty of our baby's spirit and human self, we also heal ourselves.

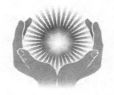

Afterword

It has been six years since I wrote the first edition of *Welcoming Consciousness*. As a core text for our prenatal and perinatal psychology graduate students, we have engaged in lively class discussions based on the material and perspective introduced in the book. What became clearer to me is that so much of what prenatal and perinatal psychology has unearthed has been the unfortunate-to-tragic consequences of what we have lost in our modern era understanding of babies. Much of what we teach has focused on early trauma and life-diminishing patterns set in motion. As in this book, many of the stories we have witnessed concern what happens when we deny babies' sentient nature and do not consider the needs of the conscious baby. Prenatal and perinatal psychology has provided us with the knowledge of what can cause physical and mental illnesses and life diminishing patterns, and we can now identify, mitigate, and therapeutically intervene to transform these even during infancy. Yet, the field has so much more to offer that needs to be articulated.

I have always admired the attachment community and how effectively they have aligned theory, research, professional practice, parenting practice and parent-to-parent support groups by articulating a core set of principles that holds what is known and valued to support healthy attachment. Although our field had already made a tremendous contribution by learning more about early development from the baby's perspective, I felt we had not yet effectively articulated our findings in ways that could act as a guide post for positive early development.

In 2007, with grant funding, we started the community organization *Natural Family Living~Right From the Start* and gathered leaders in the field of prenatal and perinatal psychology and specifically those working with babies, to develop a set of guiding principles that emerged from our findings. What principles did we believe supported human potential and optimal relationships from the beginning of life? At the core of our principles we sought to provide a lens through which to view the *continuity of early human life and relationship* from pre-conception forward, and to better understand how to support human potential and optimal relationships throughout the prenatal and infancy periods.

In 2008, we published these guiding principles, and they are available in English and Spanish at: www.naturalfamilylivingsb.org. As we go to press with our second edition of *Welcoming Consciousness*, a position paper written by myself with Dr. Marti Glenn, *Investing in Human Potential From the Beginning of Life*, is being published in the *Journal of Prenatal and Perinatal Psychology and Health* that include these principles in our recommendations.

Whereas the Integrated Model and Integrated Self are my own unique interpretations of our findings and model, these principles represent a collective voice from many in prenatal and perinatal psychology.

12 Guiding Principles To Support Human Potential and Optimal Relationships From the Beginning of Life

1. The Primary Period

The *primary period for human development* occurs from preconception through the first year of postnatal life. This is the time in which vital foundations are established at every level of being: physical, emotional, mental, spiritual and relational.

2. Forming the Core Blueprint

Experiences during this primary period form the blueprint of our core perceptions, belief structures, and ways of being in the world with others and ourselves.

- These foundational elements are implicit, observable in newborns, and initiate life-long ways of being.
- These core implicit patterns profoundly shape our being in life-enhancing or life-diminishing directions.

3. Continuum of Development

Human development is continuous from prenatal to postnatal life. Postnatal patterns build upon earlier prenatal and birth experiences.

- Optimal foundations for growth and resiliency, including brain development, emotional intelligence, and self-regulation are predicated upon optimal conditions during the pre-conception period, pregnancy, birth and the first year of life.

- Optimal foundations of secure attachment and healthy relationships are predicated upon optimal relationships during the pre-conception period, during pregnancy, the birth experience and the first year of life.

4. Capacities & Capabilities

Human beings are conscious, sentient, aware, and possess a sense of Self even during this very early primary period.

- We seek ever-increasing states of wholeness and growth through the expression of human life. This innate drive guides and infuses our human development.
- From the beginning of life, babies perceive, communicate, and learn, in ways that include an integration of mind-to-mind, energetic, and physical-sensorial capacities and ways of being.

5. Relationship

Human development occurs within relationship from the beginning. Human connections and surrounding environment profoundly influence the quality and structure of every aspect of baby's development.

- From the beginning of life, baby experiences and internalizes what mother experiences and feels. Father and/or partner's relationship with mother and baby are integral to optimizing primary foundations for baby.
- All relationships and encounters with mother, baby, and father during this primary period affect the quality of life and baby's foundation. Supportive, loving, and

healthy relationships are integral to optimizing primary foundations for baby.

6. Innate Needs

The innate need for security, belonging, love and nurturing, feeling wanted, feeling valued, and being seen as the Self we are is present from the beginning of life. Meeting these needs and providing the right environment supports optimal development.

7. Communication

Babies are continually communicating and seeking connection. Relating and responding to babies in ways that honor their multifaceted capacities for communication supports optimal development and wholeness.

8. Mother-Baby Interconnectedness

Respecting and optimizing the bond between mother and baby and the mother-baby interconnectedness during pregnancy, birth, and infancy is of highest priority.

9. Bonding

Birth and bonding is a critical developmental process for mother, baby, and father that form core patterns with life-long implications.

- The best baby and mother outcomes occur when mother feels empowered and supported and the natural process of birth is allowed to unfold with minimal intervention and no interruption in mother-baby connection and physical contact. If any separation of baby from mother occurs, continuity of father's contact and connection with baby should be supported.

- Baby responds and thrives best when the relationship with mother is undisturbed, when baby is communicated with directly, and when the process of birth supports baby's ability to orient and integrate the series of events.

10. Resolving & Healing

Resolving and healing past and current conflicts, stress, and issues that effect the quality of life for all family members is of highest priority. Doing so before pregnancy is best. When needed, therapeutic support for mother, baby, and father provided as early as possible during this vital primary period is recommended for optimal outcomes.

11. Underlying Patterns

When unresolved issues remain or less than optimal conditions and experiences occur during conception, pregnancy, birth and the first postnatal year, life diminishing patterns often underlay health issues, stress behaviors, difficulty in self-regulation, attachment, learning, and other disorders over the life-span.

12. Professional Support

These early diminishing patterns are imbedded below the level of the conscious mind in the implicit memory system, subconscious, and somatic patterns. Professionals trained in primary psychology (prenatal and perinatal psychology) can identify these patterns and support babies, children, parents and adults to heal and shift these primary patterns to more life-enhancing ones at any age. When parents resolve and heal their own unresolved issues from their child's pregnancy and birth, their children benefit at any age.

Primary Psychology

The following section is an excerpt from an article by myself and Dr. Marti Glenn, *Primary Psychology: Bridging the Divide in Early Development* (2008).

In the process of formulating the guiding principles the need for a shift in perspective that embraces the continuity of human development and relationship from prenatal to postnatal life became evident. The experiential learning, development of relationships, and the formulation of life-patterns during the prenatal period clearly demonstrate the undivided continuum of human experience from conception forward.

Prenatal and perinatal psychology has been instrumental in mapping the understanding of our prenatal, birth and bonding experiences and how they formulate our core human blueprints. We now see the need to apply this perspective to the first year of postnatal life. Although many groups demarcate birth through year three as the primary developmental period, we focus on the period from pre-conception through the first natal year. We saw a natural demarcation at the end of the first year because most of the core patterns are already established within the first months of postnatal life. And, by the infant's first birthday, the mother-baby interconnectedness naturally expands to include a larger reality as baby's abilities support further exploration of his/her larger world.

Our intention is to expand, extend, and enfold what has been known as prenatal and perinatal psychology into a discipline known as *Primary Psychology*. The vital lens of prenatal and perinatal psychology—the multifaceted view of babies and the map of how early experiences during conception, prenatal life and birth and bonding form core blueprints—lays the foundation for primary psychology. Primary psychology extends that lens and perspective through baby's first postnatal year.

The word primary means both first and most vital, and holds the essence and significance of this period of development. Thus, primary psychology focuses on the continuity of experience and development from preconception through baby's first postnatal year, and we call this period the *primary period* of human and relational development when *primary foundations* are developed.

Primary psychology is a synergy of prenatal and perinatal psychology along with other leading-edge disciplines such as biodynamic embryology, infant mental health, attachment, early trauma, developmental neurosciences, consciousness studies and other new sciences. Prenatal and perinatal psychology has revealed that babies are sentient, aware, learning, multifaceted, and capable human beings who already have a sense of Self. Clearly these findings join many of the new sciences and perspectives that suggest consciousness to be at the core of human nature, life, and healing. Be it holistic, integrative, or integral models and approaches, each speaks to a recognition of our wholeness and integrity and anchors consciousness as fundamental.

Primary psychology and the findings from prenatal and perinatal psychology illuminate consciousness at the very beginning of human life. By acknowledging the sentient, aware and communicative capacities of babies in the womb, we believe we can best meet and support the sustained integration of mind, body and spirit from the beginning of life.

Primary psychology education seeks to provide expertise for those working with young families. We recommend these

12 guiding principles to support advocacy for funding, training, clinical practice, and community programs that provide "early intervention" to support families as they prepare, conceive, carry, birth and care for their baby through the first year of postnatal life. (McCarty, W. and Glenn, M., 2007)

The New Frontiers in Primary Psychology

All that we are learning about the primary period of development and about our multidimensional nature are thrilling to me. I believe we are entering a new era, the era of supporting more connection with who we really are from the beginning of life. We now understand so much more about how important our role is in supporting consciousness during the transition from spirit to human life. Each of us can contribute to babies being more fully connected to who they really are and living their lives as *Spiritual Human Beings*.

Not only does primary psychology help us support human potential at the beginning of life, it provides us a map to understanding ourselves and clues to healing primary patterns that separate us from our fullest potential at any age.

Wishing you the best in your life,
Wendy

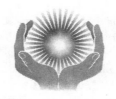

References

Beebe, B. (1998). A procedural theory of therapeutic action: commentary on the symposium, "Interventions that effect change in psychotherapy". *Infant Mental Health Journal, 19*(3), 333-340.

Carman, E. M. & Carman, N. J. (1999). *Cosmic cradle: Souls waiting in the wings for birth.* Fairfield, IO: Sunstar Publishing, Inc.

Chamberlain, D. (1988). *Babies remember birth.* Los Angeles, CA: Jeremy P. Tarcher.

Chamberlain, D. (1998). *The mind of your newborn baby* (3rd ed.). Berkeley, CA: North Atlantic Books.

Chamberlain, D. (1999a). Reliability of birth memory: Observations from mother and child pairs in hypnosis. *Journal of Prenatal and Perinatal Psychology and Health, 14*(1-2), 19-29. (Originally published in the *Journal of the American Academy of Medical Hypnoanalysts, 1*(2), 89-98, 1986).

Chamberlain, D. (1999b). The significance of birth memories. *Journal of Prenatal and Perinatal Psychology and Health, 14*(1-2), 65-84.

Dossey, L. (1999). *Reinventing medicine: Beyond mind-body to a new era of healing.* New York: HarperSanFranciso.

Dossey, L. (2003). Samueli conference on definitions and standards in healing research: Working definitions and terms. *Definitions in Healing Research, 9*(3), A10-A11.

Emerson, W. R. (1998). Birth trauma: The psychological effects of obstetrical interventions. *Journal of Prenatal & Perinatal Psychology & Health, 13*(1), 11-44.

Emerson, W. R. (1998). The vulnerable prenate. *The International Journal of Prenatal and Perinatal Psychology and Medicine, 10*(1), 5-18. (Originally published in 1998, *Journal of Prenatal & Perinatal Psychology & Health,* 10(3), 125-142.)

Emerson, W. R. (1999a). *Pre- and perinatal treatment of children and adults: Collected works II.* (Available from Emerson Training Seminars, http://www.emersonbirthrx.com)

Emerson, W. R. (1999b). Shock: A universal malady—Prenatal and perinatal origins of suffering. (Audiotapes and booklet). (Available from Emerson Training Seminars, http://www.emersonbirthrx.com)

Emerson, W. R., (2001a). Treating cesarean birth trauma during infancy and childhood. *Journal of Prenatal and Perinatal Psychology, 15*(3), 177-192.

Emerson, W. R. (2001b). *Treatment of birth trauma in infants and children: Collected works 1.* (Available from Emerson Training Seminars, http://www.emersonbirthrx.com)

Farrant, G. (1986a). *Cellular consciousness.* Keynote address at the 14th IPA Convention, August 30, 1986. Retrieved February 22, 2002, from http://webpages.charter,net/jspeyrer/gfarrant.htm.

Farrant, G. (1986b). Cellular consciousness. *Aesthema,* 7, 28-39.

Gabriel, M. (1992). *Voices from the womb.* Lower Lake, CA: Aslan Publishing.

Hallett, E. (1995). *Soul Trek: Meeting our children on the way to birth.* Hamilton, MT: Light Hearts Publishing.

Hart, Tobin (2003). *The secret spiritual world of children.* Maui, HI: Inner Ocean Publishing, Inc.

Ho, M. W. (1998, 2003). *The rainbow and the worm: The physics of organisms.* River Edge, NJ: World Scientific.

Ho, M. W. (2000). The entangled universe. *YES! A Journal of Positive Futures.* Spring, 20-23.

Houston, J. *Reality and how it works.* Retrieved August 3, 2004, from http://www.jeanhourston.org/lectures/realtiy.html.

Larimore, T. & Farrant, G. *Universal body movements in cellular consciousness and what they mean.* (Originally published in Primal Renaissance, 1:1). Retrieved April 2, 2004, from http://www/terrylarimor.com/Cellular.html.

Levine, P. (1997). *Waking the tiger: The innate capacity to transform overwhelming experience.* Berkeley, CA: North Atlantic Books.

Lewis, M. D. & Granic, I. (Eds.). (2000). *Emotion, development, and self-organization: Dynamic systems approaches to emotional development.* Cambridge, UK: Cambridge University Press.

Linn, S. & Emerson, W. & Linn D. & Linn, M. (1999). *Remembering our home: Healing hurts and receiving gifts from conception to birth.* Mahwah, NJ: Paulist Press.

Lipton, B. (2001). Nature, nurture and human development. *Journal of Prenatal and Perinatal Psychology and Health, 16*(2), 167-180.

Lipton, B. (2005). *The biology of belief: Unleashing the power of consciousness, matter, and miracles.* Santa Rosa, CA: Mountain of Love/Elite Books.

Marcer, P. J. & Schempp, W. (1997). Model of the neuron working by quantum holography. *Informatica,* 21, 519-534.

Marcer, P. J. & Schempp, W. (1998). The brain as a conscious system. *International Journal of General Systems.*

McCarty, W. A. (1996). *Being with babies: What babies are teaching us, an introduction, 1.* Goleta, CA: Wondrous Beginnings.

McCarty W. A. (1997). *Being with babies: What babies are teaching us, supporting babies' innate wisdom, 2.* Goleta, CA: Wondrous Beginnings.

McCarty, W. A. (2002a). The power of beliefs: What babies are teaching us. *Journal of Prenatal & Perinatal Psychology & Health, 16*(4), 341-360.

McCarty, W. A. and Glenn, M.A. (2009). Investing in human potential from the beginning of life: Keys to maximizing human capital. *Journal of Prenatal & Perinatal Psychology & Health (in press).*

McCarty, W. A. and Glenn, M. A. (2008). *Primary Psychology: Bridging the Divide of Early Development.* (Retrieved from www.naturalfamilylivingsb.org on 6/22/08).

McCraty, R. Bradley, R. T. & Tomasino, D. The resonance heart. *SHIFT: At the frontiers of consciousness.* December 2004-January 2005, 15-19.

McCraty, R., Atkinson, M., & Bradley, R. T. (2004). Electrophysiological evidence of intuition: Part 1. The surprising role of the heart. *The Journal of Alternative and Complementary Medicine, 10*(1), 133-143.

McCraty, R., Atkinson, M., & Bradley, R. T. (2004). Electrophysiological evidence of intuition: Part 2. A system-wide process? *The Journal of Alternative and Complementary Medicine, 10*(2), 325-336.

McTaggart, L. (2002). *The field: The quest for the secret of the universe.* New York: HarperCollins.

Mendizza, M. & Pearce, J. C. (2001). Magical parent, magical child: The optimum learning relationship. Nevada City, CA: Touch the Future. (You may obtain them directly from the publisher: www.ttfuture.org.)

Mitchell, E. *Nature's mind: The quantum hologram.* Retrieved November 22, 2003, from http://www.edmitchellapollo14.com/naturearticle.html

Natural Family Living~Right From the Start (2008). *Nurturing human potential and optimizing relationships from the beginning of life: 12 guiding principles from primary psychology.* [Brochure]. Santa Barbara, CA: http://www.naturalfamilylivingsb.org

Odent, M. (1999). *The scientification of love.* London: Free Association Books.

Pearce, J. C. (2002). *The Biology of transcendence: A blueprint of the human spirit.* Rochester, VT: Park Street Press.

Raymond, S. (1988). Cellular consciousness and conception: An interview with Dr. Graham Farrant. *Pre- & Perinatal Psychology News, 2*(2) Summer. 4-22.

Radin, D. (1997). *The conscious universe: The scientific truth of psychic phenomena.* San Francisco: HarperSanFrancisco.

Schwartz, G. & Russek, L. G. (1999). *The living energy universe.* Charlottesville, VA: Hamptom-Roads Publishing Co.

Schwartz, G. (2002). *The afterlife experiments: Breakthrough scientific evidence of life after death.* Pocket Books.

Sills, F. (2001). *Craniosacral biodynamics: The breath of life, biodynamics, and fundamental skill.* (Vol I). Berkeley, CA: North Atlantic Books.

Somé, Sobonfu E. (1999). *Welcoming spirit home: Ancient African teachings to celebrate children and community.* Novato, CA: New World Library.

Talbot, M. (1992). *The holographic universe.* New York: Harper Perennial.

Wade, J. (1996). *Changes of mind: A holonomic theory of the evolution of consciousness.* Albany, NY: State University of New York Press.

Wade, J. (1998). Physically transcendent awareness: A comparison of the phenomenology of consciousness before birth and after death. *Journal of Near-Death Studies, 16*(4), 249-275.

Stevenson, I. (2000). Unusual play in young children who claim to remember previous lives. *Journal of Scientific Exploration, 14*(4), 557-570.

Wambach, H. (1979). *Life before life.* New York: Bantam Books.

Wilber, K. (1982) (Ed.). *The holographic paradigm and other paradoxes: Exploring the leading edge of science.* Boulder, CO: Shambala Publications.

Wilber, K. (1998). *The marriage of sense and soul: Integrating science and religion.* New York: Broadway Books.

Wilber, K. (2000). *A theory of everything: An integral vision for business, politics, science and spirituality.* Boston: Shambala Publications.

Wilber, K. (2000). *Integral psychology: Consciousness, spirit, psychology, therapy.* Boston: Shambala.

Appendix
Terms and Definitions

From Dossey, L. (2003). Samueli conference on definitions and standards in healing research: Working definitions and terms. *Alternative Therapies in Health and Medicine, 9*(3) Supplement, 10-12.

Printed with permission from InnoVision Communications.

Attention: The focus of conscious awareness on an object, experience, sensation, or process.

Consciousness: The capacity to react to, attend to, and be aware of self and other. Consciousness subsumes all categories of experience, including perception, cognition, intuition, instinct, will and emotional, at all levels, including those commonly termed "consciousness," "subconsciousness," "superconsciousness," or "unconscious," "intention," and "attention," without presumption of specific psychological or physiological mechanisms. Neither consciousness nor its environment exists in isolation; they can be represented only in interaction and exchange of information. Philosophical consciousness: Philosophically, consciousness is a state or quality of being with a capacity for sentience and subjectivity. It is contrasted with being "nonconscious," a state of affairs wholly without sentience or subjectivity. Philosophical consciousness is about the context of consciousness; it is about the model of being that makes possible any and all contents of consciousness. Psychological consciousness: Psychologically, consciousness is a state of awareness characterized by being awake or alert, and is contrasted with the "unconscious," a state of being asleep, or with psychic contents below the threshold of conscious-awake awareness. Psychological consciousness is about the contents of consciousness and about the mode of access (conscious or unconscious) to these contents.

Field: A force that can cause action at a distance.

Intention: The conscious determination to do a specific thing or to act in a specific manner; the mental state of being committed to, planning to, or trying to perform an action.

Nonlocality: Generally, the state of being unconfined and unrestricted to a particular place. In modern physics, a fundamental property of the universe, in which entities once in contact demonstrate correlated behaviors, instantly and to the same degree, regardless of the extent of spatial separation. Nonlocal events are unconstrained by lightspeed and have 3 defining characteristics: they are unmediated (by any known form of physical signals), unmitigated (the degree of correlation does not diminish with increasing spatial separation), and immediate.

Spirituality: The feelings, thoughts, experiences, and behaviors that arise from a search for that which is generally considered sacred or holy. Spirituality is usually, though not universally, considered to involve a sense of connection with an absolute, imminent, or transcendent spiritual force, however named, as well as the conviction that meaning, value, direction, and purpose are valid aspects of the universe.

Transpersonal: Beyond the individual ego, mind, and body.

Transpersonal psychology: A system of personal understanding that is based on people's experiences of temporarily transcending their usual identification with their limited biological, historical, cultural, and personal self and, at the deepest and most profound levels of experience possible, recognizing/becoming something of vast intelligence and compassion that encompasses/is the entire universe. From this perspective, the ordinary, biological, historical, cultural, and personal self is seen as an important, but quite partial (and often pathologically distorted) manifestation or expression of this much greater something that is our deeper origin and destination.

Other Terms and Definitions

Sentient: responsive to or conscious of sense impressions; aware; finely sensitive in perception of feeling (Merriam Webster Online. Retrieved August 14, 2004 from http://www.m-w.com/)

Appendix
Bibliography

Category of Inquiry

Contemporary Early Development and Infancy
　　Assessment and Diagnosis
　　Attachment Theory and Research
　　Development and Developmental Theory
　　Development and Psychopathology
　　Infant Psychotherapy
　　Journals

Prenatal and Perinatal Psychology (PPN)
　　Biodynamic Embryology and Craniosacral Therapy
　　PPN Theory, Adult Patterns, and Adult Psychotherapy
　　PPN Birth and Bonding
　　PPN Prenates and Infants
　　PPN Oriented Therapeutic Work with Young Families
　　PPN Oriented Parenting
　　Journals and Resources

General Topics
　　After-Death Communication
　　Humanistic and Transpersonal
　　Wilber Material
　　Life Between Life
　　Near Death Experiences
　　Out-of-Body Experiences and Remote Viewing
　　Past Life and Reincarnation
　　Physics, World View, Holographic Theory, Holistic Healing,
　　　　and Energy Studies
　　Journals

Contemporary Early Development and Infancy

Assessment and Diagnosis

Black, M. M. and Matula, K. (1999). *Essential of Bayley scales of infant development II assessment.* New York: Wiley, John & Sons, Inc.

DeWeerd, A. W. (1995). Atlas of EEG In the First Months of Life. Departments of Clinical Neurophysiology, Juliana Children Hospital, Westeinde Hospital, The Hague, The Netherlands, 1-91.

Diagnostic classification: 0 – 3: Diagnostic classification of mental health and developmental disorders of infancy and early childhood. Washington, D.C.: ZERO TO THREE.

DeGangi, G. (2000). *Pediatric disorders of regulation in affect and behavior: A therapist's guide to assessment and treatment.* San Diego, CA: Academic Press.

Gilliam, W. S. & Mayes, L. C. (2000). Developmental assessment of the infants and toddlers. In C. H. Zeanah (Ed.), *Handbook of infant mental health,* 2nd ed. (pp. 236-248). New York: Guilford Press.

Singer, L. T. & Zeskind, P. S. (2001). *Biobehavioral assessment of the infant.* New York: The Guilford Press.

Zeanah, C. H., et al. (2000). Infant-parent relationship assessment. In C. H. Zeanah (Ed.), *Handbook of infant mental health,* 2nd ed. (pp. 236-248). New York: Guilford Press.

Attachment Theory and Research

Ainsworth, M. D. S., Blehar, M. C., Waters, E., & Wall, S. (1978). *Patterns of attachment: A psychological study of the strange situation.* Hillsdale, NJ: Lawrence Erlbaum.

Ainsworth, M. D. S. & Bowlby, J. (1991). An ethological approach to personality development. *American Psychologist, 46,* 333-341.

BelSunny, J. (2002). Developmental origins of attachment styles. *Attachment & Human Development, 4*(2), 166-170.

Bowlby, J. (2000). *Separation: Anxiety and anger.* New York: Basic Books.

Bowlby, J. (2000). *Attachment* (2nd Ed.). New York: Basic Books.

Bowlby, J. (2000). *Loss: Sadness and depression.* New York: Basic Books.

Bowlby, J. (1990). *A secure base: Parent-child attachment and healthy human development.* New York: Basic Books.

Boris, N. W. & Zeanah, C. H. (1999). Disturbances and disorders of attachment in infancy: An overview. *Infant Mental Health Journal, 20*(1), 1-9.

Cassidy, J. & Shaver, R. (Eds.) (1999). *Handbook of attachment.* New York: Guilford Press.

Cozolino, L. (2006). *The neuroscience of human relationships: Attachment and the developing social brain.* New York: W. W. Norton & Company, Inc.

Fonagy, P., Steele, H. & Steele, M. (1991). Maternal representations of attachment during pregnancy predict the organization of infant-mother attachment at one year of age. *Child Development, 62*, 891-905.

Fonagy, P. & Target, M. (1997). Attachment and reflective function: Their role in self-organization, *Development and Psychopathology, 9*, 679-700.

Fonagy, P. (2001). *Attachment theory and psychoanalysis.* New York: Other Press.

Greenberg, M. T., Cicchetti, D. & Cummings, E. M. (1990). *Attachment in the preschool years: Theory, research, and intervention.* Chicago: The University of Chicago Press.

Greenspan, S. I. (1992). *Infancy and early childhood: the practice of clinical assessment and intervention with emotional and developmental challenges.* Madison, CT: International Universities Press, Inc.

Karen, R. (1994). *Becoming attached: First relationships and how they shape our capacity to love.* New York: Oxford Press University.

Koulomzin, M., Beebe, B., Anderson, S., Jaffe, J., Feldstein, S. & Crown, C. (2002). Infant gaze, head, face and self-touch at 4 months differentiate secure vs. avoidant attachment at 1 year: A microanalytic approach. *Attachment & Human Development, 4*(1), 3-24.

Panksepp, J. (2001). The long-term psychobiological consequences of infant emotions: prescriptions for the twenty-first century. *Infant Mental Health Journal, 22*(1-2), 132-173.

Soloman, J. & George, C. (1999). *Attachment disorganization.* New York: Guilford Press.

Waters, E., Merrick, S., Treboux, D., Crowell, J. & Albersheim, L. (2000). Attachment security in infancy and early adulthood: A twenty-year longitudinal study. *Child Development, 71*(3), 684-689.

Development and Developmental Theories

This section also includes self-regulation, self-organization, memory, and sensory integration.

Aitken, K. J. & Trevarthen, C. (1997). Self/other organization in human psychology development. *Development and Psychopathology, 9*, 653-677.

Bornstein, M. H., Lamb, M. E., & Lamb, M. (2002). *Development in infancy: An introduction* (4th ed.). Lawrence Erlbaum Associates, Inc.

Bower, T. G. R. (1989). *The rational infant: Learning in infancy.* New York: W. H. Freeman and Company.

Brazelton, T. & Sparrow, J. (1992). *Touchpoints: Birth to three.* Boulder, CO: Perseus Books Group.

Bremner, G. & Fogel, A. (Eds.). (2000). *Blackwell handbook of Infant Development.* Malden, MA: Blackwell Publishers.

Call, J. D., Galenson, E., & Tyson, R. L. (Eds.). (1984). *Frontiers of infant psychiatry.* (Vol. 2). New York: Basic Books.

Davis, M., and Wallbridge. (1981). *Boundary and space: An introduction to the work of D. W. Winnicott.* London: H. Karnac Books, Ltd.

Eliot, L. (1999). *What's going on in there? How the brain and mind develop in the first five years of life.* New York: Bantum Books.

Feldman, R. (2003). Infant-Mother and Infant-Father synchrony: The coregulation of positive arousal. *Infant Mental Health Journal, 24*(1), 1-23.

Fogel, A. (2000). *Infancy: Infant, family and society* (4th ed.). Belmont, CA: Wadsworth/Thomson Learning.

Fonagy, P., Gergely, G., Jurist, E. L., & Target, M. (2002). *Affect regulation, mentalization, and the development of self.* New York: Other Press.

Fujioka, T., Fujioka, A., Endoh, H., Sakata, Y., Furukawa, S. & Nakamura, S. (2003). Materno-fetal coordination of stress-induced FOS expression in the hypothalamic paraventricular nucleus during pregnancy. *Neuroscience, 118*, 409-415.

Gaensbauer, T. J. (2002). Representations of trauma in infancy: Clinical and theoretical implications for the understanding of early memory. *Infant Mental Health Journal, 23*(3), 259-277.

Geber, M. (1958). The psycho-motor development of African children in the first year, and the influence of maternal behavior. *The Journal of Social Psychology, 47*, 185-195.

Gopnik, A., et al. (1999). *The scientist in the crib: Minds, brains and how children learn.* New York: William Morrow & Co.

Gilliam, W. S. & Mayes, L. C. (2000). In C. H. Zeanah (Ed.). *Handbook of infant mental health* (2nd ed.). (pp. 236-248). New York: Guilford Press.

Ginsburg, H. & Opper, S. (1969). *Piaget's theory of intellectual development: An introduction.* Englewood Cliffs, NJ: Prentice-Hall, Inc.

Harding, C. G., Weissmann, L., Kromelow, S. & Stillson, S. R. (1997). Shared minds: How mothers and infants co-construct early patterns of choice within intentional communication partnerships. *Infant Mental Health Journal, 18*(1), 24-39.

Hart, T. (2003). The secret spiritual world of children. Makawao, HI: Inner Ocean Publishing, Inc.

Jaffe, J., et. al. (2001). *Rhythms of dialogue in infancy.* Malden, MA: Blackwell Publishers.

Kellman, P. J. & Arterberry, M. E. (2000). *The cradle of knowledge: development of perception in infancy.* Cambridge, MA: MIT Press.

Kranowitz, C. S. (1998). *The out-of-sync child: Recognizing and coping with sensory integration dysfunction.* New York: Perigee Books.

Lewis, M. D. & Granic, I. (Eds.). (2000). *Emotion, development, and self-organization: Dynamic systems approaches to emotional development.* Cambridge, UK: Cambridge University Press.

Mahler, M. S., Pine, F., and Bergman, A. (1975). *The psychological birth of the human infant.* New York: Basic Books.

Main, M. (1995). Recent studies in attachment: overview, with selected implications for clinical work. In S. Goldberg, R. Muir & J. Kerr (Eds.), *Attachment theory: Social, developmental and clinical perspective* (pp. 407–474). Hillsdale, NJ: Analytic Press.

Muir, D. & Slater, A. (Eds.). (2000). *Infant development: The essential readings (Essential readings in developmental psychology).* Malden, MA: Blackwell Publishers.

Piontelli, A. (2000). From fetus to child: An observational and psychoanalytic study. In E. B. Spillius, *New Library of Psycholoanalysis, 15,* Philadelphia, PA: Brunner-Routledge. (Originally published in 1992, London: Routledge).

Richters, J. E. (1997). The hubble hypothesis and the developmentalist's dilemma, *Development and Psychopathology, 9,* 193-229.

Ryan, R. M., Kuhl, J., Deci, E. L. (1997). Nature and autonomy: An organizational view of social and neurobiological aspects of self-regulation in behavior and development. *Development and Psychopathology, 9,* 701-728.

Sander, L. W. (2000). Where are we going in the field of infant mental health? *Infant Mental Health Journal, 21*(1-2), 5-20.

Schore, A. N. (1994). *Affect regulation and the origin of the self.* Hillsdale, NJ:

Lawrence Erlbaum Associates.

Schore, A. N. (2001). Effects of a secure attachment relationship on right brain development, affect regulation, and infant mental health. *Infant Mental Health Journal, 22*(1-2), 7-66.

Shonkoff, J. P. & Phillips, D. A. (Eds.). (2000). *From neurons to neighborhoods: The science of early childhood development.* Washington, D.C.: National Academy Press.

Siegel, D. (1999). *The developing mind: Toward a neurobiology of interpersonal experience.* New York: The Guilford Press.

Siegel, D. J. & Hartzell, M. (2003). *Parenting from the inside out: How a deeper self-understanding can help you raise children who thrive.* New York: Jeremy P. Tarcher.

Stern, D. N. (1985). *The interpersonal world of the infant: A view from psychoanalysis and developmental psychology.* New York: Basic Books.

Stern, D. N., Bruschweiler-Stern, N., Harrison, A. M., Lyons-Ruth, K., Morgan, A. C., Nahum, J. R., Sander, L. & Tronick, E. Z. (1998). The process of therapeutic change involving implicit knowledge: Some implications of developmental observations for adult psychotherapy. *Infant Mental Health Journal, 19*(3), 300-308.

Stockholm, J. N. (2001). The psychoanalyst and the baby: A new look at work with infants. *International Journal of Psychoanalysis, 82*, 83-100.

Tronick, E. Z., Bruschweiler-Stern, N., Harrison, A. M., Lyons-Ruth, K., Morgan, A. C., Nahum, et al. (1998). Dyadically expanded states of consciousness and the process of therapeutic change. *Infant Mental Health Journal, 19*(3), 290-299.

Tronick, E. (2007). *The neurobehavioral and social-emotional development of infants and children.* New York: W. W. Norton & Company, Inc.

Wheeler, M. A., Stuss, D. T. & Tulving, E. (1997). Toward a theory of episodic memory: The frontal lobes and autonoetic consciousness. *Psychological Bulletin, 121*(3), 331-354.

Winnicott, D. W. (1971). *Playing and reality.* London: Tavistock Publications

Winnicott, D. W. (1987). *The child, the family and the outside world.* Reading, MA: Addison-Wesley Publishing Co.

Winnicott, D. W. (1987). *Babies and their mothers.* Reading, MA: Addison-Wesley Publishing Co.

Winnicott, D. W. (1988). Human nature. New York: Schocken Books.

Zeanah, C. H., et al. (1993) (Eds.). *Handbook of infant mental health.* New York: Guilford Publications, Inc.

Zeanah, C. H., et al. (2000) (Eds.). *Handbook of infant mental health* (2nd ed.). New York: Guilford Publications, Inc.

Development and Psychopathology

Cicchetti, D. & Richters, J. E. (1997). Examining the conceptual and scientific underpinnings of research in developmental psychopathology. *Development and Psychology, 9,* 189-191.

Jameson, P. B., Gelfand, D. M., Kulcsar, E. & Teti, D. M. (1997). Mother-toddler interaction patterns associated with maternal depression. *Development and Psychology, 9,* 537-550.

Jones, N. A., Field, T., Fox, N. A., Lundy, B. & Davalos, M. (1997). EEG activation in 1-month-old infants of depressed mothers. *Development and Psychopathology, 9,* 491-505.

Schore, A. N. (1997). Early organization of the nonlinear right brain and development of a predisposition to psychiatric disorders. *Development and Psychopathology, 9,* 595-631.

Schore, A. N. (2001). The effects of early relational trauma on right brain development, affect regulation, and infant mental health. *Infant Mental Health Journal, 22*(1-2), 201-269.

Schore, A. N. (2002). Dysregulation of the right brain: A fundamental mechanism of traumatic attachment and the psychopathogenesis of posttraumatic stress disorder. *Australian and New Zealand Journal of Psychiatry, 36,* 9-30.

Schore, A. N. (2003). *Affect regulation and the repair of the self.* New York: W.W. Norton & Company.

Schore, A. N. (2003). *Affect dysregulation and disorders of the self.* New York: W.W. Norton & Company.

Infant Psychotherapy (and a few on adults)

Baradon, T. (2002). Psychotherapeutic work with parents and infants—psychoanalytic and attachment perspectives. *Attachment & Human Development, 4*(1), 25-38.

Beebe, B. (1998). A procedural theory of therapeutic action: commentary on the symposium, "interventions that effect change in psychotherapy". *Infant Mental Health Journal, 19*(3), 333-340.

Beebe, B. (2003). Brief Mother-Infant treatment: Psychoanalytically informed video feedback. *Infant Mental Health Journal, 24*(1), 24-52.

Beebe, B. & Lachmann, F. M. (2002) *Infant research and adult treatment.* Hillsdale,

NJ: The Analytic Press.

Cohen, N. J., et al.(1999). Watch, wait, and wonder: Testing the effectiveness of a new approach to mother-infant psychotherapy. *Infant Mental Health Journal 20*(4), 429-451.

Cohen, N. J., et al. (2002). Six-month follow-up of two mother-infant psychotherapies: Convergence of therapeutic outcomes. *Infant Mental Health Journal, 23*(4), 361-380.

Fonagy, P. (1998). Prevention, the appropriate target of infant psychotherapy. *Infant Mental Health Journal, 19*(2), 124-150.

Heinicke, C. M., et al. (2000). Relationship-based intervention with at-risk mothers: Factors affecting variations in outcome. *Infant Mental Health Journal, 21* (3), 133-55.

Levine, P. A. & Kline, M. (2007). *Trauma through a child's eyes: Awakening the ordinary miracle of healing.* Berkeley, CA: North Atlantic Books.

Lieberman, A. F., & Zeanah, C. H. (1999). Contributions of attachment theory to infant-parent psychotherapy and other interventions with infants and young children. In J. Cassidy & P. R. Shaver (Eds.), *Handbook of attachment* (pp. 555-574). New York: Guildford Press.

Lieberman, A. F. & Van Horn, P. (2008) *Psychotherapy with infants and young children.* New York: The Guilford Press.

Lojkasek, M., Cohen, N. J. & Muir, E. (1994). Where is the infant in infant intervention? A review of the literature on changing troubled mother-infant relationships. *Psychotherapy, 31*(1), 208-220.

Mahrer, A. R., Levinson, J. R. & Fine, S. (1976). Infant psychotherapy: Theory, research, and practice. *Psychotherapy, 13*(2), 131-140.

Minde, K. & Hesse, E. (1996). The role of the adult attachment interview in parent-infant psychotherapy: A case presentation. *Infant Mental Health Journal, 17*(2), 115-126.

OsofSunny, J. D. (2004). *Young children and trauma: Intervention and treatment.* New York: Guilford Press.

Robert-Tissot, C., Cramer, B., Stern, D. N., Rusconi Serpa, S., Bachmann, J. P., Palacio-Espasa, F., et al. (1996). Outcome evaluation in brief mother-infant psychotherapies: Report on 75 cases. *Infant Mental Health Journal, 17*(2), 97-114.

Sander, L., Bruschweiler-Stern, N., Harrison, A. M., Lyons-Ruth, K., Morgan, A. C., Nahum, J. R., et al. (1998). Interventions that effect change in psychotherapy: A model based on infant research. *Infant Mental Health Journal, 19*(3), 280-281.

Stockholm, J. N. (2001). The psychoanalyst and the baby: A new look at work with infants. *International Journal of Psychoanalysis, 82,* 83-100.

Williamson, G. G. & Anzalone, M. E. (2001). Sensory integration and self-regulation in infants and toddlers: Helping very young children interact with their environment. Washington, D.C.: ZERO TO THREE.

Journals and Resources

Advances in Infant Research (Book Series)
Alternative Therapies
American Scientist
Attachment & Human Development
Birth
Child Abuse Review
Child Development
Child Development Abstracts
Development and Psychopathology
Developmental Psych Abstracts
Developmental Psychobiology
Developmental Psychology
Early Development and Parenting
Infancy
Infant and Child Development
Infant Behavior and Development
Infant Mental Health Journal
Infant Observation Journal
Infants and Young Children
Journal of Child Psychology and Psychiatry
Journal of Clinical Child Psychology
Journal of Counseling & Clinical Psychology
Journal of Genetic Psychology
Journal of Obstetrics and Gynecology
Journal of Reproductive and Infant Psychotherapy
International Society on Infant Studies
Books of the Society for Research in Child Development
Progress in Infancy Research (Book series)
Psychological Medicine
Psychiatry
Science

Journals and Resources (Continued)

For a more complete list of journals in the developmental neurosciences, psychiatry, and psychoanalytic perspectives, see the extensive reference sections in Allan Schore's texts.

NCAST: Nursing Child Assessment Satellite Training, www.ncast.org
Parent-infant interaction assessments, feeding and teaching assessments, states of consciousness, etc.
www.waimh.org - World Association for Infant Mental Health
www.ttfuture.org - Touch the Future
www.zerotothree.org
www.Attach.org

Prenatal and Perinatal Psychology (PPN)

The PPN bibliography section primarily focuses on certain aspects within the field of prenatal and perinatal psychology and does not represent the breadth of the field. Areas such as pregnancy and birth, prenatal intervention programs, prenatal factors and outcome, prevention programs, and more birth-oriented articles are not represented below.

Biodynamic Embryology and Craniosacral Therapy

Blechschmidt, E. (2004). *The ontogenetic basis of human anatomy: A biodynamic approach to development from conception to birth.* (B. Freeman, Trans.). Murrieta, CA: Pacific Distributing.

Blechschmidt, E. & Gasser, R. (1978). *Biokinetics and biodynamics of human differentiation.* Springfield, IL: Charles C. Thomas Publisher.

Frymann, V. (1966). Relation of disturbances of craniosacral mechanism to symptomatology of the newborn: Study of 1,250 infants. *Journal AOA, 65,* 1059-1075.

Kern, M. (2001). *Wisdom in the body: The craniosacral approach to essential health.* London: Thorsons.

Shea, M. (2002). *Biodynamic craniosacral therapy: A primer.* North Palm Beach, FL: Shea Educational Group.

Sills, F. (2001). *Craniosacral biodynamics: The breath of life, biodynamics, and fundamental skill.* (Vol 1). Berkeley, CA: North Atlantic Books.

Sills, F. (2004). *Craniosacral biodynamics: The primal midline and the organization of the body.* (Vol 2). Berkeley, CA: North Atlantic Books.

PPN: Theory, Adult Patterns, and Adult Psychotherapy

Armstrong, T. (1988). *The radiant child.* Wheaton, Ill: Quest Books.

Axness, M. W. (2001). Toward a fluid dance in seamless dress: The field of pre- and perinatal development challenges researchers to integrate scientific and spiritual orientations. *Journal of Prenatal & Perinatal Psychology & Health, 16*(2), 135-149.

Axness, M. (2004). Malattachment and the self struggle. *Journal of Prenatal and Perinatal Psychology and Health, 19*(2), 131-147.

Bache, M. (2000). *Dark night, early dawn.* Albany, NY: State University of New York Press.

Blazy, H. (1998). The European discoveries in prenatal ethnology and archeology of the Mind. *The International Journal of Prenatal and Perinatal Psychology and Medicine, 10*(4), 429-438.

Blazy, H. (1996). The psychoanalytic and the prenatal "partnership". *The International Journal of Prenatal and Perinatal Psychology and Medicine Suppl., 8,* 39-46.

Bongard, J. (2000). *The near birth experience: A journey to the center of self.* New York: Marlowe and Company.

Chamberlain, D. B. (1990). Expanding the boundaries of memory. *Pre- and Peri-natal Psychology, 4*(3), 171-189.

Chamberlain, D. B. (1999). Foundations of sex, love and relationships: From conception to birth. *Journal of Prenatal and Perinatal Psychology and Health, 14*(1-2), 45-64.

Chamberlain, D. B. (1999). Prenatal body language: A new perspective on ourselves, *Journal of Prenatal and Perinatal Psychology and Health, 14*(1-2), 169-186.

Chamberlain, D. B. (1999). Reliability of birth memory: observations from mother and child pairs in hypnosis, *Journal of Prenatal and Perinatal Psychology and Health, 14*(1-2), 19-30.

Chamberlain, D. B. (1999). The significance of birth memories. *Journal of Prenatal and Perinatal Psychology and Health, 14 (1-2), 65-84.*

Chamberlain, D. B. (1999). Transpersonal adventures in prenatal and perinatal hypnotherapy. *Transpersonal Hypnosis.* FL: CRC Press.

Chamberlain, D. B. (2001). *Vanishing Twin Syndrome* (In Psychotherapy: Repatterning Techniques Panel). 10th International Congress of The Association of Prenatal and Perinatal Psychology and Health. San Francisco. (Available through Gold Key Recordings: vgoldkey@evl.net)

Cheek, D. B. (1974). Sequential head and shoulder movements appearing with age regression in hypnosis to birth. *American Journal of Clinical Hypnosis, 16*(4), 261-266.

Cheek, D. B. (1993). Are telepathy, clairvoyance and 'hearing' possible in utero? Suggestive evidence as revealed during hypnotic age-regression studies of prenatal memory. *Pre- and Perinatal Psychology Journal, 7*(2), 125-138.

Cheek, D. B. (1986). Prenatal and perinatal imprints: Apparent prenatal consciousness as revealed by hypnosis. *Pre- and Perinatal Psychology Journal, 1*(2), 97-110.

Costa Segui, M. (1995). The prenatal period as the origin of character structures. *The International Journal of Prenatal and Perinatal Psychology and Medicine, 7*(3), 309.

Culbert-Koehn, J. (1999). Prenatal and perinatal influences in contemporary Jungian analysis. *The International Journal of Prenatal and Perinatal Psychology and Medicine, 11*(3), 277-286.

deMause, L. (1982). *Foundations of psychohistory*. New York: Creative Roots, Inc.

deMause, L. (1996). Restaging fetal traumas in war and social violence. *The International Journal of Prenatal and Perinatal Psychology and Medicine, 8*(2), 171-212.

Dosh, M. A. (1999). Prenatal and perinatal foundations of moral development. *Journal of Prenatal & Perinatal Psychology & Health, 13*(3-4), 213-222.

Emerson, W. R. (1998). Birth trauma: The psychological effects of obstetrical interventions. *Journal of Prenatal & Perinatal Psychology & Health, 13*(1), 11-44.

English, J. B. (1985). Different doorway: Adventures of a caesarean born. Point Reyes Station, CA: Earth Heart.

English, J. B. (1993). Being born caesarean: Physical, psychological and metaphysical aspects. *Pre- and Perinatal Psychology Journal, 7*(3), 215-230.

Farrant, G. (1986a). *Cellular consciousness.* Keynote address at the 14th IPA Convention, August 30, 1986. Retrieved February 22, 2002, from http://webpages.charter,net/jspeyrer/gfarrant.htm.

Farrant, G. (1986b). Cellular consciousness. *Aesthema, 7,* 28-39.

Fedor-Freybergh, P. (1993). Prenatal psychology and medicine: A new approach to primary prevention. *The International Journal of Prenatal and Perinatal Psychology and Medicine, 5*(3), 285-292.

Findeisen, B. R. (1993). Pre- and perinatal losses. *Pre- and Perinatal Psychology Journal*, *8*(1), 65-77.

Gabriel, M. ((1992). *Voices from the womb*. Lower Lake, CA: Aslan Publishing.

Grof, S. (1985). *Beyond the brain: Birth death, and transcendence in psychotherapy.* Albany, NY: State University of New York Press.

Grof, S. (1988). *The adventures in self-discovery.* Albany, NY: State University of New York Press.

Grof, S. (2000). *Psychology of the future: Lessons from modern consciousness research.* Albany, NY: State University of New York Press.

Ham, J. T. & Kilmo, J. (2000). Fetal Awareness of maternal emotional states during pregnancy. *Journal of Prenatal and Perinatal Psychology and Health* *15*(2), 118-145.

Herskowitz, M. (1996). Wilhelm Reich: Studies of earliest childhood. *The International Journal of Prenatal and Perinatal Psychology and Medicine, 8*(4), 415-426.

Hollenweger, J. (1993). Prenatal development and the structure of experience. *The International Journal of Prenatal and Perinatal Psychology and Medicine, 5*(3), 293-302.

House, S. H. (1999). Primal integration therapy–school of Lake. *The International Journal of Prenatal and Perinatal Psychology and Medicine, 11*(4), 437-458.

Hull, W. F. (1986). Psychological treatment of birth trauma with age regression and its relationship to chemical dependency. *Pre- and Perinatal Psychology Journal, 1(2)*, 111-134.

Ingalls, P. M. S. (1996). Birth memories, psychotherapy, and philosophy. *The International Journal of Prenatal and Perinatal Psychology and Medicine, 8*(2), 157-170.

Ingalls, P. M. S. (1997). Birth traumas: Violence begets violence. *The International Journal of Prenatal and Perinatal Psychology and Medicine, 9*(2), 181-196.

Ingalls, P. M. S. (2001). Born to live. Part 2: A care history. *International Journal of Prenatal and Perinatal Psychology and Medicine, 13*(3-4), 223-239.

Irving, M. (1997). Sexual assault and birth trauma: Interrelated issues. *Pre- and Peri-natal Psychology Journal, 11*(4), 215-250.

Irving-Neto, R. L. & Verny, T. R. (1992). Pre- and perinatal experiences and personality: A retrospective analysis. *Pre- and Perinatal Psychology Journal, 7*(2), 139-172.

161

Jacobson, B. (1988). Perinatal origin of eventual self-destructive behavior. *Pre- and peri-natal psychology, 2*(4), 227-241.

Jacobson, B. (2000). Obstetrical care and proneness of offspring to suicide as adults: A case-control study. *Journal of Prenatal and Perinatal Psychology and Health, 15(1), 63-74.*

Janov, A. (1983). *Imprints: The lifelong effects of the birth experience.* New York: Coward McCann, Inc.

Janus, L. (1997). *The enduring effects of prenatal experience: Echoes from the womb.* (T. Dowling, Trans.). Northdale, NJ: Jason Aronson Inc.

Janov, A. (2000). *The biology of love.* Amherst, New York: Prometheus Books.

Kafkalides, Z. (2002). Prenatal environment and postnatal life in S. Grof's, F. Lake's and A. Kafkalides' work. *The International Journal of Prenatal and Perinatal Psychology and Medicine, 14*(1-2), 9-18.

Lapidus, L. B. (1991). Cross-cultural consistencies in prenatal perceptual patterns and perinatal practices. *The International Journal of Prenatal and Perinatal Studies, 3*(3-4), 155-168.

Larimore, T. & Farrant, G. *Universal body movements in cellular consciousness and what they mean.* (Originally published in *Primal Renaissance,1*:1). Retrieved April 2, 2004, from http://www.terrylarimore.com/cellular.html

Lipton, B. (1998). Nature, nurture, and the power of love. *Journal of Prenatal & Perinatal Psychology & Health 13*(1), 3-10.

Lipton, B. (2001). Nature, nurture and human development. *Journal of Prenatal and Perinatal Psychology and Health, 16*(2), 167-180.

Lyman, B. J. (1999). Antecedents to somatoform disorders: A pre- and perinatal psychology hypothesis. *Journal of Prenatal and Perinatal Psychology and Health, 13*(3-4), 247-254.

Lyman, B. J. (2008). Prenatal and perinatal trauma case formulation: Toward an evidence-based assessment of the origins of repetitive behaviors in adults. *Journal of Prenatal and Perinatal Psychology and Health 22*(3), 189-218.

Lyman, B. J. (2005). Prenatal and perinatal psychotherapy with adults: An integrative model for empirical testing. *Journal of Perinatal and Perinatal Psychology and Health, 20*(1), 58-77.

MacLean, C. A. (2003). Transpersonal dimensions in healing trauma of the unborn child. *Journal of Prenatal & Perinatal Psychology & Health, 17*(3), 203-223.

MacLean, C. A. (2003). Transpersonal dimensions in healing pre/perinatal trauma with EMDR (eye movement desensitization and reprocessing. *Journal of Prenatal and Perinatal Psychology and Health, 18*(1), 39-70.

Maiwald, M. & Janus, L. (1993). Development, behavior and psychic experience in the prenatal period and the consequences for life history – a bibliographic survey. *The International Journal of Prenatal and Perinatal Psychology and Medicine, 5*(4), 451.

Maret, S. M. (1997). *The prenatal person: Frank Lake's maternal-fetal distress syndrome.* New York: University Press of America.

Marquez, A. (2000). Healing through prenatal and perinatal memory recall: A phenomenological investigation. *Journal of Prenatal and Perinatal Psychology and Health, 15(2)* 146-172.

Menzam, C. (2002). *Dancing Our Birth: Prenatal and Birth Themes and Symbols in Dance, Movement, Art, Dreams, Language, Myth, Ritual, Play, and Psychotherapy.* Unpublished dissertation. Union Institute and University.

Moss, R. C. (1986). Frank Lake's maternal-fetal distress syndrome and primal integration workshops. Part 2. *Pre- and Peri-natal Psychology Journal, 1(1)* 52-68.

Nobel, E. (1993) *Primal Connections: How our experience from conception to birth influences our emotions, behavior and health.* Fireside, NY: Penguin Books.

Prescott, J. W. The origins of human love and violence. *Pre- and Peri-natal Psychology Journal, 10*(3), 143—188.

Ray, S. & Mandel, B. ((1987). *Birth and relationships: How your birth affects your relationships. Berkeley,* CA: CelestralArts.

Raymond, S. (1987). Prenatal memories as a diagnostic psychothera-peutic tool. *Pre- and Perinatal Psychology Journal, 1*(4), 3003-317.

Raymond, S. (1988). Cellular consciousness and conception: An interview with Dr. Graham Farrant. *Pre- & Perinatal Psychology News,2*(2) Summer.

Renggli, F. (2003). Tracing the Roots of Panic to Prenatal Trauma. *Journal of Prenatal and Perinatal Psychology and Health 17*(4), 289-300.

Renggli, F. (2005). Healing and birth. *Journal of Prenatal and Perinatal Psychology and Health 19*(4), 303-318.

Righetti, P. L. (1996). The emotional experience of the fetus: A preliminary report. *Journal of Prenatal & Perinatal Psychology & Health, 11*(1), 55-65.

Riley, C. D. (1986). Tess: The emotional and physiological effects of prenatal physical trauma. *Journal of Pre-and Perinatal, 1*(1), 69-74.

Schier, K. (2001). The prenatal trauma in families of children with anorexia nervosa and bronchial asthma. *The International Journal of Prenatal and Perinatal Psychology and Medicine, 13*(3-4), 213-222.

Seelig, M. (1998). Re-experiencing pre- and perinatal imprints in non-ordinary states of consciousness. *The International Journal of Prenatal and Perinatal Psychology and Medicine, 10*(3), 323-342.

Segui, M. C. The prenatal period as the origin of character structures. *International Journal of Prenatal and Perinatal Psychology and Medicine, 7*(3), 309-322.

Share, L. (1996). Dreams and the reconstruction of infant trauma. *The International Journal of Prenatal and Perinatal Psychology and Medicine, 8*(3), 295-316.

Sjezer, M. & Barbier, C. (2000). Reflections on the notion of traumatism at birth. *The International Journal of Prenatal and Perinatal Psychology and Medicine, 12*(1), 127.

Sonne, J. C. (1994). The relevance of the dread of being aborted to models of therapy and models of the mind. Part II: Mentation and communication with the unborn. *The International Journal of Prenatal and Perinatal Psychology and Medicine, 6*(2), 247-275.

Sonne, J. C. (1996). Interpreting the dread of being aborted in therapy. *The International Journal of Prenatal and Perinatal Psychology and Medicine, 8*(3), 317-340.

Sonne, J. C. (1998). Psychoanalytic perspectives of adoption. *The International Journal of Prenatal and Perinatal Psychology and Medicine, 10*(3), 295-312.

Sonne, J. C. (1994). The relevance of the dread of being aborted to models of therapy and models of the mind. Part I: Case examples. *The International Journal of Prenatal and Perinatal Psychology and Medicine, 6*(1), 67-86.

Sonne, J. C. (2001). It's proven but not believed. An exploration of psychosocial resistances to acceptance of the reality of prenatal mentation, communication, and psychic trauma. *The International Journal of Prenatal and Perinatal Psychology and Medicine, 13*(1-2), 43-82.

Sonne, J. C. (2002). The varying behaviors of fathers in the prenatal experience of the unborn: Protecting, loving and "welcoming with arms wide open," vs. ignoring, unloving, competitive, abusive, abortion-minded or aborting. *The International Journal of Prenatal and Perinatal Psychology and Medicine, 14*(1-2), 33-52.

Sonne, J. C. (2005). The varying behaviors of fathers in the prenatal experience of the unborn: Protecting, loving, and "welcoming with arms wide open," vs. ignoring, unloving, competitive, abusive, abortion minded or aborting. *Journal of Prenatal and Perinatal Psychology and Health, 19*(4), 319-340.

Turner, J. R. (1988). Birth, life and more life: Reactive patterning based on prebirth events. In Fedor-Freybergh, P. G. & Vogel, M. L. V. (Eds.). *Prenatal and perinatal psychology and medicine, encounter with the unborn: A comprehensive survey of research and practice* (pp. 309-316). NJ: Parthenon Publishing Group.

Turner, J. R. & Turner, T. G.. (1993). Prebirth memory therapy, including prematurely delivered patients. *Pre- and Perinatal Psychology Journal, 7*(4), 321-332.

Turner, J. R. & Turner, T. G. (2003). Violence and pregnancy: A whole-self psychology perspective. *Journal of Prenatal and Perinatal Psychology and Health, 17*(4), 301-320.

Turner, J. R., Turner, T., & Westermann, S. (1999). Prebirth memory discovery in psychotraumatology. *The International Journal of Prenatal and Perinatal Psychology and Medicine, 11*(4), 469-486.

Verny, T. R. (1989). The scientific basis of pre-and perinatal psychology, part I. *Pre- and Perinatal Psychology Journal, 3*(3), 157-170.

Verny, T. R. (1994). Working with pre- and perinatal material in psychotherapy. *The International Journal of Prenatal and Perinatal Psychology and Medicine, 8*(3), 161-186.

Verny, T. R. (1996). Isolation, Rejection and Communion in the Womb. *The International Journal of Prenatal and Perinatal Psychology and Medicine, 8*(3), 287-294.

Verny, T. R. (Ed.) (1987). *Pre- and Peri-natal Psychology: An introduction.* New York: Human Sciences Press, Inc.

Wade, J. (1996). *Changes of mind: A holonomic theory of the evolution of consciousness.* Albany, New York: State University of New York Press.

Wade, J. (1998). Physically transcendent awareness: A comparison of the phenomenology of consciousness before birth and after death. *Journal of Near-Death Studies, 16*(4), 249-275.

Wambach, H. (1979). *Life before life.* New York: Bantam Books.

Wilheim, J. (1992). The emergence of early prenatal traumatic imprints in psychoanalytic practice – from preconception to birth. *The International Journal of Prenatal and Perinatal Studies, 4*(3-4), 179-186.

Wilheim, J. (1998). Clinical manifestations of traumatical imprints. *The International Journal of Prenatal and Perinatal Psychology and Medicine, 10*(2), 153-162.

Wilheim, J. (2002). Cellular memory: clinical evidence. *The International Journal of Prenatal and Perinatal Psychology and Medicine, 14*(1-2), 19-32.

Winnicott, D. W. (1992). Birth memories, birth trauma and anxiety. *The International Journal of Prenatal and Perinatal Studies, 4*(1-2), 17-34.

Zimberoff, D. & Hartman, D. (1998). Insidious trauma caused by prenatal gender prejudice. *Journal of Prenatal & Perinatal Psychology & Health, 13*(1), 45-51.

PPN: Birth and Bonding

Arms, S. (1994). *Immaculate deception II: A fresh look at childbirth.* Berkeley, CA: Celestrial Arts.

Baker, J. P. (1996). Shamanic midwifery–every mother a midwife. *The International Journal of Prenatal and Perinatal Psychology and Medicine, 8*(1), 15-20.

Buckley, S. J. (2005). *Gentle birth, gentle mothering.* Brisbane, Australia: One Moon Press.

Davis-Floyd, R. E. (1990). Obstetrical rituals and cultural anomaly: Part I. *Pre- and Peri-natal Psychology Journal, 4*(3), 193-211.

Davis-Floyd, R. & Sargent, C. F. (1997). *Childbirth and authoritative knowledge: Cross-cultural perspectives.* Berkeley, CA: University of California Press.

Goer, H. (1995). *Obstetrical myths versus research realities: A guide to the medical literature.* Westport, CT: Bergin & Garvey.

Karll, S. (2003). *Sacred birthing: Birthing a new humanity.* Victoria, Canada: Trafford Publishing.

Klaus, M. & Kennell, J. (1982). *Parent infant bonding.* St. Louis: Mosby.

Klaus, M., Kennell, J., & Klaus, P. H. (1995). *Bonding: Building the foundations of secure attachment and independence.* Cambridge: Perseus.

Klaus, M. & Klaus, P. H. (1998). *Your amazing newborn.* Cambridge: Perseus.

Newman, R. (2005). *Calm birth: New method for conscious childbirth.* Berkeley, CA: North Atlantic Books.

Odent, M. (1999). *The scientification of love.* London: Free Association Books.

Odent, M. (2004). *The caesarean.* London: Free Association Books.

Rand, M. L. (1999). As it was in the beginning: The significance of infant bonding in the development of self and relationships. *The International Journal of Prenatal and Perinatal Psychology and Medicine, 11*(4), 487-494.

Righard, L. & Alade, M. O. (1990). Effect of delivery room routines on success of first breast-feed. *Lancet, 336,* 1105-1107.

PPN: Prenates and Infants

Adamson-Macedo, E. N. (1998). The mind and body of the preterm neonate. *The International Journal of Prenatal and Perinatal Psychology and*

Medicine, 10(4), 439-456.

Attree, J. L. A. & Adamson-Macedo, E. N. (1998). Assessing early memories of youngsters born pre-term: A follow-up study. *The International Journal of Prenatal and Perinatal Psychology and Medicine, 10*(1), 39.

Brekhman, G. I. & Smirnov, K. K. (2001). Water as energoinformative connection channel between an unborn child, its mother and environment. *The International Journal of Prenatal and Perinatal Psychology and Medicine, 13*(1-2), 93-98.

Carman, E. M. & Carman, N. J. (1999). *Cosmic cradle: Souls waiting in the wings for birth.* Fairfield, IO: Sunstar Publishing, Inc.

Chamberlain, D. B. (1990). The expanding boundaries of memory. *Pre- and Peri-Natal Psychology, 4*(3), 171-189.

Chamberlain, D. B. (1992). Babies are not what we thought: Call for a new paradigm. *The International Journal of Prenatal and Perinatal Studies, 4*(3-4), 161-178.

Chamberlain, D. B. (1993). How pre- and perinatal psychology can transform the world. *The International Journal of Prenatal and Perinatal Psychology and Medicine, 5*(4), 413-424.

Chamberlain, D. B. (1994). The sentient prenate: What every parent should know. *Pre- and Peri-natal Psychology Journal, 9*(1), 9-34.

Chamberlain, D. B. (1998). Prenatal receptivity and intelligence. *Journal of Prenatal & Perinatal Psychology & Health, 12*(3-4), 95-117.

Chamberlain, D. (1998). *The mind of your newborn baby.* Berkeley, CA: North Atlantic Books.

Chamberlain, D. B. (1999). Babies don't feel pain: A century of denial in medicine. *Journal of Prenatal & Perinatal Psychology & Health, 14*(1-2), 145-168.

Chamberlain, D. B. (2000). Prenatal body language: A new perspective on ourselves. *The International Journal of Prenatal and Perinatal Psychology and Medicine, 12*(4), 541-556.

Cheek, D. B. (1992). Are telepathy, clairvoyance and "hearing" possible in utero? Suggestive evidence as revealed during hypnotic age-regression studies of prenatal memory. *Pre- and Perinatal Psychology Journal, 7*(2), 125-137.

Church, D. (1988). *Communicating with the spirit of your unborn child.* San Leandro, CA: Aslan Publishing.

Coplan, R. J., O'Neil, K., & Arbeau, K. A. (2005). Maternal anxiety during and after pregnancy and infant temperament at three months of age.

Journal of Prenatal and Perinatal Psychology and Health, 19(3), 199-216.

Eichhorn, D. & Verny, T. R. (1999). The biopsychosocial transactional model of development: The beginning of the formation of an emergent sense of self in the newborn. *Journal of Prenatal & Perinatal Psychology & Health, 13*(3-4), 223-234.

Emerson, W. R. (1998). The vulnerable prenate. *The International Journal of Prenatal and Perinatal Psychology and Medicine, 10*(1), 5-18.

Engler-Hicks, B. (2007). The alchemical dance of mother and infant: A blueprint for co-creative dyadic unity during the prenatal and perinatal period. *Journal of Prenatal and Perinatal Psychology and Health 22*(1), 5-30.

Field, T., et al., (2002). Prenatal anger effects on the fetus and neonate. *Journal of Obstetrics & Gynaecology, 22*(3): 260-266.

Gilliland, A. L. & Verny, T. R. (1999). The effects of domestic abuse on the unborn child. *Journal of Prenatal & Perinatal Psychology & Health, 13*(3-4), 235-245.

Hallet, E. (1995). *Soul trek: Meeting our children on the way to birth.* Hamilton, MT: Light Hearts Publishing.

Hallett, E. (2002). *Stories of the unborn soul: The mystery and delight of pre-birth communication.* San Jose: Writers Club Press.

Ikegawa, A. (2002). *I remember when I was in mommy's tummy* (K. K. Bondet & S M Smith, Trans.). Chiyoda-ky, Tokyo: Lyons Co. Ltd.

Jones, C. (1989). *From parent to child: The psychic link.* New York: Warner Books. Northvale, NJ: Jason Aronson, Inc.

Little, J. F. & Hepper, P. G. (1995). The psychological effects of maternal smoking on fetal movements. *The International Journal of Prenatal and Perinatal Psychology and Medicine, 7*(2), 161-167.

McCarty, W. A. (2007). Editorial. Special issue: Doctoral research. *Journal of Prenatal and Perinatal Psychology and Health, 22*(1), 1-3. (Guest editor for journal issue).

Nesci, D. A., Poliseno, T. A., Averna, S., Mancuso, A. K., Ancona, L., Ferrazzani, S., et al. (1993). The "covert" relationship between mother and her unborn child. *The International Journal of Prenatal and Perinatal Psychology and Medicine, 5*(2), 169-176.

Nesci, D. A., Poliseno, T. A., Averna, S., Mancuso, A. K., Ancona, L. & Mancuso, S. (1996). Ultrasound research on prenatal life: Transcripts of a clinical experience. *The International Journal of Prenatal and Perinatal Psychology and Medicine, 8*(2), 139-144.

Panuthos, C. (1983). The psychological effects of cesarean deliveries.

Mothering, 61-72.

Piontelli, A. (2000). *From fetus to child.* Philadelphia, PA: Brunner-Routledge.

Piontelli, A. (2002). Twins: *From fetus to child.* Philadelphia, PA: Brunner-Routledge.

Pomeroy, W. (1995). A working model for trauma: The relationship between trauma and violence, *Pre- and Peri-natal Psychology Journal, 10*(2), 89-102.

Raffai, J. (1998). Mother-child bonding-analysis in the prenatal realm: The strange events of a queer world. *The International Journal of Prenatal and Perinatal Psychology and Medicine, 10*(2), 163-174.

Takikawa, D. (Director & Producer). 2004. *What babies want.* [Documentary film]. (Available from www.whatbabieswant.com)

Thompson, P. (2004). The impact of trauma on the embryo and fetus: An application of the diathesis-stress model and the neurovulnerability-neurotoxicity model. *Journal of Prenatal and Perinatal Psychology and Health, 19*(1), 9-64.

PPN-Oriented Therapeutic Work with Young Families

Blasco, T. M. (2007). Prenatal and perinatal memories in preverbal children: Clinical observations using videotape examination. *Journal of Prenatal and Perinatal Psychology and Health 22*(1), 31-54.

Castellino, R. (1995). *The polarity therapy paradigm regarding pre-conception, prenatal and birth imprinting.* (Available from Castellino Training Seminars, (805) 687-2897).

Castellino, R. (2000). The stress matrix: Implications for prenatal and birth therapy. *Journal of Prenatal and Perinatal Psychology and Health, 15*(1), 31-62.

Castellino, R. (1997). *The caregiver's role in birth and newborn and self-attachment needs.* Santa Barbara, CA: BEBA. (Available from BEBA, (805) 687-2897).

Emerson, W. R. (2001a). Treating cesarean birth trauma during infancy and childhood. *Journal of Prenatal and Perinatal Psychology, 15*(3), 177-192.

Emerson, W. R. (2001b). *Treatment of birth trauma in infants and children: Collected works 1.* (Available from Emerson Training Seminars, http://www.emersonbirthrx.com)

Emerson, W. R. (1999). *Pre- and perinatal treatment of children and adults: Collected works II.* (Available from Emerson Training Seminars, http://www.emersonbirthrx.com)

Emerson, W. R. (1999). Shock: A universal malady–Prenatal and perinatal origins of suffering. (Audiotapes and booklet). (Available from Emerson Training Seminars, http://www.emersonbirthrx.com)

LaGoy, L. (1993). The loss of a twin in utero's affect on pre-natal and post-natal bonding. *The International Journal of Prenatal and Perinatal Psychology and Medicine, 5*(4), 439-444.

Lubetzky, O. (2001). A glimpse into the world of an extremely low-birth-weight, prematurely born infant: Case study of a 10-year-old boy. *The International Journal of Prenatal and Perinatal Psychology and Medicine, 13*(3-4), 241 -246.

McCarty, W. A. (1996). *Being with babies: What babies are teaching us, an introduction, 1.* Goleta, CA: Wondrous Beginnings.

McCarty W. A. (1997). *Being with babies: What babies are teaching us, supporting babies' innate wisdom, 2.* Goleta, CA: Wondrous Beginnings.

McCarty, W. A. (2002). The power of beliefs: What babies are teaching us. *Journal of Prenatal & Perinatal Psychology & Health, 16*(4). 341-360.

McCarty, W. A. (2002) Keys to healing and preventing foundational trauma: What babies are teaching us. *Bridges—ISSSEEM Magazine, 13*(4), 8-12.

McCarty, W. A. (2004). The CALL to reawaken and deepen our communication with babies: What babies are teaching us. *International Doula, 12*(2), Summer 2004.

McCarty, W. A. (2005). Nurturing the Possible: Supporting the integrated self from the beginning of life. *Shift: At the Frontiers of Consciousness* 6, 18-20.

McCarty, W. A. (2006). Supporting babies' wholeness in the 21st century: An integrated model of early development. *Journal of Prenatal & Perinatal Psychology & Health, 21*(2), 187-220.

McCarty, W. A. (2006) Clinical story of a 6-year-old boy's eating phobia: An integrated approach utilizing prenatal and perinatal psychology with energy psychology's emotional freedom technique (EFT) in a surrogate non-local application. *Journal of Prenatal & Perinatal Psychology & Health, 21(2), 117-139.*

McCarty, W.A. (2007). EFT for Mom, baby, and dad from the beginning of life. Chapter in *15 Ways to Health, Happiness, and Abundance.* Ebook available at www.tryitoneverything.com

Szejer, M. (2005). Talking to babies: healing with words on a maternity ward (J. M. Todd, Trans.). Boston: Beacon Press.

Ward, S. A. Birth Trauma in Infants and Children. *Journal of Prenatal & Perinatal Psychology & Health, 13*(3-4), 201-212.

PPN-Oriented Parenting

Chamberlain, D. B. (1997). Early and very early parenting: New territories. *Journal of Prenatal & Perinatal Psychology & Health, 12* (2), 51-59.

Church, D. (1988). *Communing with the spirit of your unborn child: A practical guide to intimate communication with your unborn or infant child.* San Leandro, CA: Aslan Publishing.

Hallett, E. (1995). *Soul trek: Meeting our children on the way to birth.* Hamilton, MT: Light Hearts Publishing.

Heinicke, C. M., et al. (2000). Relationship-based intervention with at-risk mothers: Factors affecting variations in outcome. *Infant Mental Health Journal, 21*(3), 133-155.

Huxley, L. & Ferrucci, P. (1987). *The child of your dreams.* Minneapolis, MN: CompCare Publishers.

Linn, S., Emerson, W., Linn D., & Linn, M. (1999). *Remembering our home: Healing hurts and receiving gifts from conception to birth.* Mahwah, NJ: Paulist Press.

Luminare-Rosen, C. (2000*). Parenting begins before conception: A guide to preparing body, mind, and spirit for you and your future child.* Rochester, VT: Healing Arts Press.

McCarty, W. A. (1996). *Being with babies: What babies are teaching us, an introduction, 1.* Goleta, CA: Wondrous Beginnings. (Available from http//www.wondrousbeginnings.com)

McCarty W. A. (1997). *Being with babies: What babies are teaching us, supporting babies' innate wisdom, 2.* Goleta, CA: Wondrous Beginnings. (Available from http//www.wondrousbeginnings.com)

McCarty, W. A. (2004). The CALL to reawaken and deepen our communication with babies: what babies are teaching us. *International Doula 12*(2), Summer 2004. (Available from http//www.wondrousbeginnings.com)

McCarty, W. A. (2007). Wondrous beginnings with Wendy Anne McCarty, PhD, RN. *What Babies Want Audio Lecture, Vol II* [CD]. Los Olivos, CA: Hana Peace Works.

McCarty, W.A. (2008). Mother-baby bonding during pregnancy: A legacy of love. *New York Guide to Healthy Birth 2008.* New York: Choices in Childbirth.

Mendizza, M. & Pearce, J. C. (2001). Magical parent, Magical child: The optimum learning relationship. Nevada City, CA: Touch the Future (Available from publisher: www://ttfuture.org.)

Pearce, J. C. (1977). *Magical child*. New York: Bantum Books.

Pearce, J. C. (2002). *The Biology of transcendence: A blueprint of the human spirit*. Rochester, VT: Park Street Press.

Riley, C. M. (1988). Teaching mother-fetus communication: A workshop on how to teach pregnant mothers to communicate with their unborn children. *Journal of Prenatal & Perinatal Psychology & Health, 3*(2), 77-86.

Solter, A. J. (2001). *The aware baby*. Goleta, CA: Shining Star Press.

Solter, A. J. (2001). Hold me! The importance of physical contact with infants. *Journal of Prenatal & Perinatal Psychology & Health, 15*(3), 193-205.

Verny, T. (1981/1986). *The secret life of the unborn child*. New York: Dell.

Verny, T. & Weintraub, P. (2002). *Tomorrow's baby: The art and science of parenting from conception through infancy*. New York: Simon and Shuster.

Wirth, F. (2001). *Prenatal parenting: The complete psychological and spiritual guide to loving your unborn child*. New York: HarperCollins.

Journals and Resources

There are two primary journals in the PPN field:

Journal of Prenatal & Perinatal Psychology & Health (1997-present)
Pre- and Peri-natal Psychology (former name 1986 - 1997)
The International Journal of Prenatal and Perinatal Psychology and Medicine (1993-present)
The International Journal of Prenatal and Perinatal Studies
(former name 1989 - 1993)

For further information:
www.birthpsychology.com
www.isppm.de/jour_eng.html
www.birthworks.org/primalhealth/databank.phtml
www.sbgi.edu

General Topics

After-Death Communication

Altea, R. (1995). *The eagle and the rose*. New York: Warner Books.

AA-EVPNEWS. (1997) American association of electronic voice phenomena, Inc. 15 (4). Available through Sarah Estep at (410) 573-0873

Barnes, M. S. (1945). *Long distance calling: A record of other world communication through automatic writing*. New York: The William-Fredrick Press.

Contact: a triannual report of technical spirit communication research. (1996), *Continuing Life Research, 96*(3). Boulder, CO: SLR.

Guggenheim, B. & Guggenheim, J. (1995). Hello from heaven! *A new field of research—after-death communication confirms that life and love are eternal*. New York: Bantam Books.

Kubis, P. & Macy, M.(1995). *Conversations beyond the life with departed friends & colleagues by electronic means*. Boulder, CO: Griffin Publishing.

Locher, T. & Harsch-Fischbach, M.(1997) *Breakthroughs in technical spirit communication*. Boulder, CO: Continuing Life Research.

Macy, M. (2001). *Miracles in the storm: Talking to the other side with the new technology of spiritual contact*. New York: New American Library.

Martin, J. & Romanowski, P. (1994). *Our children forever: George Anderson's messages from children on the other side*. New York: Berkeley Books.

Moody, R. with Perry, P. (1993). *Reunions: Visionary encounters with departed loved ones*. New York: Villard Books.

Schwartz, G., et al. (2002). *The afterlife experiments: Breakthrough scientific evidence of life after death*. New York: Pocket Books.

Van Praagh, J. (1997). *Talking to heaven: A medium's message of life after death*. New York: Pengiun Books.

Van Praagh, J. (1999). *Reaching to heaven: A spiritual journey through life and death*. New York: Penguin Books.

Humanistic and Transpersonal Psychology

Grof, S. (1985). *Beyond the brain: Birth, death and transcendence in psychotherapy*. Albany, NY: State University of New York Press.

Grof, S. (2000). *Psychology of the future: Lessons from modern consciousness research*. Albany, NY: New York State University Press.

Maslow, A. H. (1999). *On the psychology of being*. New York: John Wiley & Sons.

Maslow, A. H. (1987). *Motivation and personality*. New York: Harper CollinsPublishers.

Pearce, J. C. (2002). *The biology of transcendence: A blueprint of the human spirit*. Rochester, VT: Park Street Press.

Smith, H. (1976). *Forgotten Truth: The common vision of the world's religion*. New York: HarperCollins.

Wade, J. (1996). *Changes of mind: A holonomic theory of the evolution of consciousness*.

Albany, NY: New York State University Press.

Wade, J. (1997). Idealizing the Cartesian-Newtonian paradigm physics on psychological theory. *Poznan Studies in the Philosophy of the Sciences and the Humanities, 56*, 9-34.

Wade, J. (1998). Physically transcendent awareness: A comparison of the phenomenology of consciousness before birth and after death. *Journal of Near-Death Studies, 16*(4), 249-275.

Walsh, R. & Vaughan, F. (Eds.). (1993). *Paths beyond ego: The transpersonal vision.* New York: Jeremy P. Tarcher/Putnam.

Wilber Material

This list is in the order of the *original* publication dates.

Wilber, K. (1993). *The spectrum of consciousness.* (2nd ed.). Wheaton, IL: Quest. (Original work published 1977)

Wilber, K. (2001). No *boundary: Eastern and western approaches to personal growth.* Boston: Shambala Publications, Inc. (Original work published 1979)

Wilber, K. (1996). *The Atman Project: A transpersonal view of human development.* Wheaton, IL: Quest. (Original work published 1980)

Wilber, K. (1982) (Ed.). *The holographic paradigm and other paradoxes: Exploring the leading edge of science.* Boulder, CO: Shambala Publications.

Wilber, K. (2001). *Eye to eye: The quest for the new paradigm* (3rd ed.). Boston: Shambala Publications. (Original work published in 1983)

Wilber, K., Engler, J., & Brown, D. P. (1986). *Transformations of consciousness: Conventional and contemplative perspectives on development.* Boston: Shambala Publications.

Wilber, K. (2000). *Grace and grit: spirituality and healing in the life and death of Treya Killiam Wilber* (2nd ed.). Boston: Shambala Publications. (Original work published in 1991)

Wilber, K. (1998). *The Essential Ken Wilber: An introductory reader.* Boston: Shambala Publications.

Wilber, K. (2001). *The eye of spirit: An integral vision for a world gone slightly mad.* Boston: Shambala Publications. (Original work published 1998)

Wilber, K. (2000). *A brief history of everything* (2nd ed.). Boston: Shambala Publications. (Original work published 1998)

Wilber, K. (1998). *The marriage of sense and soul: Integrating science and religion.* New York: Broadway Books.

Wilber, K. (2000). *Integral psychology: Consciousness, spirit, psychology, therapy.*

Boston: Shambala.

Wilber, K. (2000). *A theory of everything: An integral vision for business, politics, science and spirituality.* Boston: Shambala Publications.

Wilber, K. (2003). Kosmic Consciousness. (Audio Recording). Boulder, CO: Sounds True.

Life Between Life

Borgia, A. (1993). *Life in the world unseen.* Midway, UT: M.A.P

Borgia, A. (1956, 1988) *More about life in the world unseen.* London: Psychic Press, LTD.

Borgia, A. (2000). *Here and hereafter.* Midway, UT: M.A.P

Newton, M. (1994/2000). *Journey of souls: Case studies of life between lives.* St. Paul, MN: Llewellen Publications.

Richelieu, P. (1953). *A soul's journey.* San Francisco, CA: The Aquarian Press.

Whitton, J. L. & Fisher, J. (1986). *Life between life: Scientific exploration into the void separating one incarnation from the next.* New York: Warner Books, Inc.

White, S. E. (1940). *The Unobstructed Universe.* New York: E. P. Dutton & Co., Inc.

Near-Death Experiences

Atwater, P. M. H. (1999). *Children of the third millennium: Children's near-death experience and the evolution of humankind.* New York: Three Rivers Press.

Atwater, P. M. H. with Morgan, D. (2000). *The complete idiot's guide to near-death experiences.* Indianapolis, IN: Alpha Books/Macmillan.

Eadie, B. (1992). *Embraced by the light.* Placeville, CA: Gold Leaf Press.

Moody, R. (1975). *Life after life.* Covington, GA: Mockingbird Books.

Morse, M. with Perry, P. (1990). *Closer to the light: Learning from the near-death experiences of children.* New York: Ivy Books.

Morse, M. (2000). *Where God lives: The science of paranormal and how our brains are linked to the universe.* New York: HarperCollins Publishers, Inc.

Ring, K. (1980). *Life at death: A scientific investigation of the near-death experience.* New York: Coward, McCann and Geoghegan.

Ring, K. & Cooper, S. (1999). *Mindsight: Near-death and out-of-body experiences in the blind.* Palo Alto, CA: William James Center for Consciousness Studies.

Out-of-Body Experiences and Remote Viewing

McMoneagle, J. (1993*). Mind trek: Exploring consciousness, time, and space through* *remote viewing.* Norfolk, VA: Hampton Roads Publishing Company, Inc.

Monroe, R. A. (1971). *Journeys out of body.* New York: Doubleday.

Monroe, R. A. (1985). *Far journeys.* New York: Doubleday.

Monroe, R. A. (1994). *Ultimate journeys.* New York: Doubleday.

Past Life and Reincarnation

Bowman, C. (1997). *Children's past lives: How past life memories affect your child.* New York: Bantam Books.

Bowman, C. (2000). *Return from heaven: Reincarnation within your family.* New York: HarperCollins.

Moody, R. A. (1992). *Coming back: A psychiatrist explores past-life journeys.* New York: Bantam Books, Inc.

Stevenson, I. (1997). *Where reincarnation and biology intersect.* Westport, CT and London: Praeger.

Stevenson, I. (2000). Unusual play in young children who claim to remember previous lives. *Journal of Scientific Exploration, 14*(4), 557-570.

Wade, J. (1998). The phenomenology of near-death consciousness in past-life regression therapy: A pilot study. *Journal of Near-Death Studies, 17*(1), 3-53.

Physics, World View, Holographic Theory, Holistic Healing, and Energy Studies

Astin, J. A., Harkness, E., & Ernst, E. (2000). The efficacy of "distant healing": A systematic review of randomized trials. *Ann Intern Med., 132,* 903-910.

Beck, D. E. & Cowan, C. C. (1996). *Spiral dynamics: Mastering values, leadership and change.* Madden, MA: Blackwell Publishing.

Benford, M. S. Empirical evidence supporting macro-scale quantum holography in nonlocal effects. *Journal of Theoretics.* Retrieved August 3, 2004, from http://www.journaloftheoretics.com/Articles/2-5/Benford.htm

Benor, D. (1993). *Healing research.* Munich: Helix Verlag.

Benson, H. (1996). *Timeless healing: The power and biology of belief.* New York: Simon and Schuster.

Bohm, D. (1980). *Wholeness and implicate order.* London: Routledge and Kegan Paul.

Bohm, D. (1998). *On creativity.* (Ed. by Lee Nichol). New York: Routledge.

Bohm. D. & Hiley, B. J. (Eds.). (1995). *The undivided universe.* London:

Routledge and Kegan Paul.

Braud, W. (2003). *Distant mental influence: Its contributions to science, healing, and human interactions.* (Studies in Consciousness/Russell Targ Editions Series). Charlottesville, VA: Hampton Roads Publishing Company, Inc.

Brenner, P. (2002). *Buddha in the waiting room: Simple truths about health, illness, and healing.* Hillsborro, OR: Beyond Words Publishing, Inc.

Cha, K. Y., Wirth, D. P. & Lobo, R. A. (2001). Does prayer influence the success of in-vitro Fertilization–Embryo Transfer? Report of a masked, randomized trial [Electronic version]. *Journal of Reproduction Medicine, 46*(9).

Childre, D. and Martin, H. (1999). *The HeartMath solution.* New York: HarperSanFranciso.

Chopra, D. (1990) *Quantum healing: Exploring the frontier of mind-body medicine.* New York: Bantam Books.

Church, D. (2007). *The genie in your genes: Epigenetic Medicine and the new biology of intention.* Santa Rosa, CA: Elite Books.

Cymatics: The healing nature of sound. [video] Available through MACROmedia, (603) 659-2929.

Dossey, L. (1989). *Recovering the soul: A scientific and spiritual search.* New York: Bantam Books.

Dossey, L. (1993). *Healing words: The power of prayer and the practice of medicine.* New York: HarperCollins.

Dossey, L. (1999). *Reinventing medicine: Beyond mind-body to a new era of healing.* New York: HarperSanFranciso.

Dossey, L. (2001). *Distant intentionality and healing.* Retrieved October 8, 2001, from http:/www.emergentmind.org/Research%20Leads/_resleads/00000016.html

Dossey, L. (2003). Samueli conference on definitions and standards in healing research: Working definitions and terms. *Definitions in Healing Research, 9*(3), A10-A11.

Emoto, M. (1999). *Messages from water.* (Vol 1). Tokyo: HADO Kyoikysha CO., LTD

Emoto, M. (2001). *Messages from water.* (Vol 2). Tokyo: HADO Kyoikysha CO., LTD

Gallo, F. P. (2000). *Energy diagnostic and treatment methods.* New York: Norton.

Gerber, R. (2000). *Vibrational medicine for the 21ˢᵗ century.* New York: Harper Collins Publishers, Inc.

Goldner, D. (1999). *Infinite grace: Where the worlds of science and spiritual healing meet.* Charlottesville, VA: Hampton Roads Publishing Co., Inc.

Goswami, A. (1993). *The self-aware universe: How consciousness creates the material world.* New York: Jeremy P. Tarcher/Putnam.

Greene, B. (1999). *The elegant universe.* New York: Vintage Books.

Gribbin, J. (1984). *In search of Schrodinger's cat: Quantum physics and reality.* New York: Bantum Books.

Griffin, D. R. (1997). *Parapsychology, philosophy, and spirituality: A postmodern exploration.* Albany, NY: New York State University.

Harrison, G. M. (1999). Long-distance intercessory prayer: Personality factors of the prayor and the prayee and their effect on college success of the prayee (Doctoral dissertation, Spaulding U., 1999). *Dissertation Abstracts International, 60* (4-B) 1853.

Hart, T., Nelson, P. L. & Puhakka, K. (Eds.). (2000). *Transpersonal knowing: Exploring the horizon of consciousness.* Albany, NY: State University of New York Press.

Ho, M. W. (1998, 2003). *The rainbow and the worm: The physics of organisms.* New Jersey: World Scientific.

Ho, M. W. (2000). The entangled universe. *YES! A Journal of Positive Futures.* Spring, 20-23.

Houston, J. *Reality and how it works.* Retrieved August 3, 2004 from http://www.jeanhourston.org/lectures/realtiy.html.

Hunt, V. (1995). *Infinite mind: The science of human vibrations.* Malibu, CA: Malibu Publishing Co.

Jahn, R., Dunne, B., Bradish, G., Dobyns, Y., Lettieri, A. & Nelson, R. (2000). Mind/machine interaction consortium: PortREG replication experiments. *Journal of Scientific Exploration, 14*(4), 499-555.

Jahn, R. G. (2001). 20th and 21st century science: Reflections and projections. *Journal of Scientific Exploration, 15*(1), 21-31.

Jealous, J. (1997). Healing and the natural world. *Alternative Therapies, 3*(1), 68-76. Katra, J. & Targ, R. (1999). *The heart of the mind: How to experience god without belief.* Novato, CA: New World Library.

Lawrence, T. (1993). Bringing in the Sheep: A meta-analysis of sheep/goat experiments. In M. J. Schlitz (Ed.). *Proceedings of Presented Papers: Thirty-sixth Annual Parapsychological Association Convention.* Fairhaven, MA: Parapsychological Association.

Laszlo, E. (1995). *The interconnected universe.* Singapore: World Scientific Pub. Co., Inc.

Lazaris (1988). *The sacred journey: You and your higher self.* Orlando, CA: NPN

Publishing, Inc.

Lazaris (1996). *The Sirius Connection*. Orlando, CA: NPN Publishing, Inc.

Marcer, P. J. & Schempp, W. (1996). A mathematically specified template for DNA and the genetic code in terms of the physically realizable process of quantum holography. In Fedorec, A.M. & Marcer, P. J. (Eds.). *Proceedings of The Greenwich Symposium on Living Computers*, (pp. 45-62).

Marcer, P. J. & Schempp, W. (1997). Model of the neuron working by quantum holography. *Informatica, 21,* 519-534.

Marcer, P. J. & Schempp, W. (1998). The brain as a conscious system. *International Journal of General Systems.*

McCraty, R. (Ed). (2001). *Science of the heart: Exploring the role of the heart in human performance.* Boulder Creek, CA: HeartMath Research Center.

McCraty, R. (2003*). Heart-brain neurodynamics: The making of emotions.* Boulder Creek, CA: Institute of HeartMath.

McCraty, R. (2003). *The energetic heart: Bioelectromagnetic interactions within and between people.* Boulder Creek, CA: Institute of HeartMath.

McCraty, R., Atkinson, M., & Bradley, R. T. (2004). Electrophysiological evidence of intuition: Part I. The surprising role of the heart. *The Journal of Alternative and Complimentary Medicine, 10*(1), 133-143.

McCraty, R., Atkinson, M., & Bradley, R. T. (2004). Electrophysiological evidence of intuition: Part 2. A system-wide process. *The Journal of Alternative and Complimentary Medicine, 10*(2), 325-336.

McCraty, R., Atkinson, M., & Tomasino, D. (2003). *Modulation of DNA conformation by heart focused intention.* Boulder Creek, CA: Institute of HeartMath.

McCraty, R. & Childre, D. (2003). *The appreciative heart: The psychophysiology of positive emotions and optimal functioning.* Boulder Creek, CA: Institute of HeartMath.

McTaggart, L. (2002). *The field: The quest for the secret of the universe.* New York: HarperCollins.

Mitchell, E. *Nature's mind: The quantum hologram.* Retrieved November 22, 2003, from http://www.edmitchellapollo14.com/naturearticle.html

Mindel, A. (2000). *Quantum mind: The edge between physics and psychology.* Portland, OR: Lao Tse Press.

Newton, M. (1994, 1998). *Journey of souls: Case studies of life between lives.* St. Paul, MN: Llewellyn Publications.

Nichol. L. (1998). *On creativity: David Bohm.* New York: Routledge.

Oschman, J. L. (2002). *Energy medicine: The scientific basis.* New York: Churchill

Livingstone.

Paddison, S. (1993). *The hidden power of the heart: Discovering an unlimited source of intelligence.* Boulder, CO: Planetary Publications.

Peat, F. D. (1987). *Synchronicity: The bridge between matter and mind.* New York: Bantom Books.

Pearsall, P. (1998). *The heart's code: Tapping the wisdom and power of our heart's code.* New York: Broadway Books.

Pert, C. B. (1997). *Molecules of emotions: Why you feel the way you feel.* New York: Scribner.

Radin, D. (1997). *The conscious universe: The scientific truth of psychic phenomena.* San Francisco: HarperSanFrancisco.

Rossi, E. L. (2000). *Dreams, consciousness, spirit: The quantum experience of self-reflection and co-creation.* Malibu, CA: Palisades Gateway Publishing.

Russek, L. G. & Schwartz, G. E. (1996). Energy cardiology: A dynamical energy systems approach for integrating conventional and alternative medicine. *Advances: The Journal of Mind-Body Health, 12*(4), 4-24.

Schwartz, G. & Russek, L. G. (1997). Dynamical energy systems and modern physics: Fostering the science and spirit of complementary and alternative medicine. *Alternative Therapies, 3*(3), 46-56.

Schwartz, G. & Russek, L. G. (1999). *The living energy universe.* Charlottesville, VA: Hamptom-Roads Publishing Co.

Schiltz, M. & Braud, W. (1997). Distant intentionality and healing: Assessing the evidence. *Alternative Therapies, 3* (6), 62-73.

Schiltz, M. Amorok, T., & Micozzi, M. S. (Eds.). (2005). Consciousness & healing. *Integral approaches to mind-body medicine.* St. Louis, MO: Elsevier Churchill Livingston.

Senge, P., Scharmer, C. O., Jaworski, J., & Flowers, B. S. (2004). *Presence: Human purpose and the field of the future.* Cambridge, MA: The Society for Organizational Learning.

Sheldrake, R. (1988). *The presence of the past: Morphic resonance and the habits of nature.* New York: TimesBooks.

Sheldrake, R. (1995). *A new science of life: The hypothesis of morphic resonance.* Rochester, Va: Park Street Press.

Sheldrake, R. (1999). *Dogs that know when their owners are coming home and other unexplained powers of animals.* New York: Three Rivers Press.

Sills, F. (2001). *Craniosacral biodynamics. Vol. 1: The breath of life, biodynamics, and fundamental skills.* Berkeley, CA: North Atlantic Books.

Smith, W. L. The human electromagnetic energy field: Its relationship to interpersonal communication. *Journal of Theoretics, 4*(2) Retrieved November 25, 2004, from http://www.journaloftheoretics.com/Articles/4-2/Smith.html

Springer, S. & Eicher, D. J. (1999). Effects of a prayer circle on a moribund premature infant. [Electronic version]. *Alternative Therapies in Health and Medicine, 5*(2), 116-118.

Talbot, M. (1993). *Mysticism and the new physics.* Middlesex, England: Arkana.

Talbot, M. (1992). *The holographic universe.* New York: Harper Pernennial.

Targ, R. & Katra, J. (1999). *Miracles of mind: Exploring nonlocal consciousness and spiritual healing.* Novato, CA: New World Library.

Tiller, W. (1997). *Science and human transformation: Subtle energies, intentionality and consciousness.* Walnut Creek, CA: Pavior Publishing.

Tiller, W. A., Dibble, W. E., & Kohane, M. J. (2001). *Conscious acts of creation: The emergence of a new physics.* Pavior Publishing.

Walker, E. H. (2000). *The physics of consciousness: quantum minds and the meaning of life.* Cambridge, MA: Perseus Books.

Weil, A. (2001). On integrative medicine and the nature of reality. *Alternative Therapies, 7*(4), 97-104.

Wilson, T. D. (2002). *Strangers to ourselves: Discovering the adaptive unconscious.* Cambridge, Mass: The Belknap Press of Harvard University Press.

Wordsworth, C. *Introductory talk & demonstration on Holographic Repatterning.* [Video]. Holographic Repatterning Association. (Available from http://www.hrsalesusa.com)

Zukav, G. (1979). *The dancing wu li masters: An overview of the new physics.* New York: William Morrow & Co., Inc.

Journals

Advances in Mind-Body Medicine
Alternative Therapies in Health and Medicine
Journal of the American Society for Psychical Research
Journal of Consciousness Studies
Journal of Near-Death Studies
Journal of Scientific Exploration
Shift–Institute of Noetic Science

Appendix
The Power of Beliefs:
What Babies Are Teaching Us

McCarty, W. A. (2002). The power of beliefs: What babies are teaching us. *Journal of Prenatal & Perinatal Psychology & Health, 16*(4). 341-360.

This earlier journal article provides informative clinical stories of work with young infants from a prenatal and perinatal psychology orientation.

*This paper is based on a presentation to the 10th International Congress of APPPAH held in San Francisco, Dec. 2001. She is the founding Chair, and member of the founding faculty of the Prenatal and Perinatal Psychology Program at Santa Barbara Graduate Institute. In addition, she was the co-founder of BEBA, a non-profit clinic for therapeutic work with babies and their families. Dr. McCarty would like to thank the families whose stories are included in this paper for their participation and for permission to share their stories. Correspondence can be sent to: wmccarty@wondrousbeginnings.com.

ABSTRACT: This paper explores the development of beliefs during the prenatal and perinatal period and how babies portray their beliefs. Four vignettes from therapeutic work with babies illustrate the powerful impact beliefs already have in shaping their lives. Basic principles to help babies shift potentially constrictive beliefs to more life enhancing ones are included. This paper is intended as a theoretical and clinical exploration leading to new thought, research and clinical direction. This paper calls for a paradigm for infant development and communication with babies based on the premise that consciousness is *the* organizing principle of human experience. The importance of both practitioner and parent's beliefs is discussed.

(Clarification added 12/1/04: *Consciousness as the organizing principle.* I was developing this concept at the time of this paper, yet the way I expressed it in this paper was vague. I want to clarify that I am speaking of the primary consciousness of the person. Further evolution and articulation of this concept is found in *Welcoming Consciousness.*)

Introduction

Since I began working with children and babies within the prenatal and perinatal psychology framework in the 1980s, I have been fascinated with how *the blueprint of core beliefs* is already actively shaping babies' lives in terms of their physical structure, physiology, their relationship to self, others, and to the world as well.

The purpose of this paper is to explore the development of beliefs during the prenatal and perinatal period and how babies portray their beliefs. The importance of the practitioner and parent's beliefs is discussed. Four vignettes from therapeutic work with babies are included to illustrate the power of beliefs in babies' lives and to highlight basic principles to help babies heal and shift from potentially constrictive beliefs to more life enhancing ones. The vignettes included give babies an opportunity to teach us themselves. This paper is intended to serve as a theoretical and clinical exploration and points to new arenas of thought, research and clinical direction. This paper calls for a paradigm for infant development and communication with babies based on the premise that consciousness is *the* organizing principle of human experience. It is not intended to be a thorough examination of clinical work with babies.

About Beliefs

Our beliefs are the foundation of organization of our reality. Beliefs organize and determine what we make real. They not only shape our perception of ourselves and the world, but they continue their cascading impact by shaping and directing where we focus our attention, our motives, attitudes, thoughts, feelings, choices, decisions and our actions (Talbot, 1991; Benson, 1996). Beliefs directly impact our mental and physical health (Rossi, 1993). They are the raw materials from which our reality is created shaping our expectations of the future; they direct where we focus our most precious human treasure—our imagination. We know that much of our experience is actually filtered out before we even are aware of it. Beliefs determine what we will become conscious of or perceive.

We know that our beliefs not only filter our perceptions of reality (Ornstein and Sobel, 1987), they can even override physical reality (Rossi, 1993; Talbot, 1991). Dr. Herbert Benson (1996) in *Timeless Healing: The Power and Biology of Belief* writes of a research study in which women who had persistent nausea and vomiting during pregnancy were given a drug, syrup of ipecac, a substance that causes vomiting (Wolf, 1950). The women were told the drug would cure their problem. What happened? If physiology had the most power, the women should have continued vomiting. In fact, their vomiting stopped. Their beliefs overrode the physiological action of the drug. Benson suggests that many successful outcomes of new medical and pharmaceutical interventions reveal more about the impact of belief than about the usefulness of a specific agent. He points to three contributing factors: the belief and expectancy of the patient, the belief and expectancy of the caregiver, and the beliefs and expectancies generated by both caregiver and patient sharing similar beliefs and expectancies.

We also know that the brain cannot differentiate between what is experienced as real in the outer world and the imagined inner world. We are familiar with this in hypnosis, lucid dreaming, meditation, and other altered states in which the mind creates a reality beyond the physical outer reality (Talbot, 1991).

New research relating to babies adds to this picture. We now know that from the onset of brain wave activity and continuing throughout infancy, the delta and theta EEG ranges are predominant (Bell & Fox, 1994; Laibow, 1999). These states are associated with restorative and regenerative processes, deep creativity, hyper-learning and hypnotic suggestibility (Laibow, 1999; Robbins, 2000). Such high-voltage, slow-wave brain wave patterns are also associated with meditation, expanded awareness, psi perceptions and abilities and transcendental states of consciousness (Talbot, 1991; Wade, 1996; Wilbur, 2000).

Dr. Bruce Lipton, a cellular biologist, suggests that beliefs are *the* determining factor in whether the cellular activity is growth-oriented or protection-oriented. He proposes that prenates and babies learn at the level of perceptions. These early learned perceptions have a profound affect upon the baby's physiology and behavior and become hard-wired synaptic pathways as core perceptions becoming *subconscious beliefs* through which all later experience is filtered and organized (Lipton 1998, 2001).

When we consider the impact of shared beliefs and expectations between an adult physician and patient, the fact that the brain cannot differentiate between the imagined world and the physical world in these altered states, and realize that babies live in such altered states of deep suggestibility and learning, we must reconsider the magnitude of potential impact the beliefs and expectancies of parents and caregivers on the growing prenate and baby. We must also deepen our appreciation of the importance of our own beliefs and expectations as practitioners and parents, for it is the perceiver's beliefs that not only largely determine what is perceived, conceived and experienced when interacting with babies, but that babies are learning and associating with those beliefs when in contact with us. The enormous power of beliefs is becoming evident.

My Evolving Beliefs and Paradigm

My own perceptions in this arena have evolved over the years. During my training in obstetrical nursing and infant development during the 1970's, I was taught to look at prenates and babies through the eyes of a Newtonian model that focuses on our physically based development and experience. We examined what babies were capable of based on their brain and growing body and built our interventions based on these understandings. Behaviors that appeared outside a Newtonian-based paradigm were commonly dismissed as random or lost in the characterization as "Babies just do that. It doesn't mean anything." Although infant development theory and research has advanced greatly, and the advent of brain imagery studies has expanded our knowledge immensely in the intricacies of factors in development, the biologically based Newtonian paradigm is still predominant in infant development theory and research today.

I was first introduced to prenatal and perinatal psychology at the 1989 Pre- and Perinatal Psychology Conference in Newport Beach, CA. In his presentation there, William Emerson (1989a) included videos of his therapeutic work with babies. I was deeply moved by the baby's presence and awareness. I was stunned by this pioneering work of trauma resolution (Emerson, 1989b) during *infancy* and began to train with him.

When I entered the field of prenatal and perinatal psychotherapy with children and later with babies, my previously held beliefs and education were inadequate to explain what babies showed me each day. Was I to dismiss a four-year-old boy accurately playing out a scene from when he was five months in the womb because it could not be explained within current models? Was I to dismiss the meaningfulness of a thirteen-month old adopted boy picking a plastic character doll (out of hundreds of toys) that looked eerily like a photo of *his* birth mom the last day he saw her when he was two weeks old? Was I to disregard a three-month old girl's portrayal of the patterns, movements, and unique progression of her own birth as her parents talk of her birth? I could not dismiss what they were showing me; I was too moved by their integrity and purity of expression.

Every session with children and babies stretched my beliefs about who we are and what is possible. They were already expressing so much of their earlier experience and learned expectations of the future—if only I could hold the meaning of what they were showing me. These experiences led me to search for a paradigm to hold them. I found a home for them in a synergy of quantum physics, holographic theory, consciousness studies, transpersonal psychology, and ultimately in my own spirituality and experience as I reawakened to my own prenatal and birth experiences.

I now believe that for us to more fully and accurately understand the experience and development of the growing prenate and baby, we must acknowledge and hold a higher truth. We are consciousness prior to and beyond our physical body and brain. Within the quantum physics paradigm, consciousness is viewed as primary and thus directs and forms a partnership with our growing biology and human self (Bohm, 1980). Early experiences in the womb and during infancy appear to be an inseparable, intertwining experience between both the nonphysical realm from which we come and the physical life to which we are being initiated (Carman & Carman, 1999; Luminaire-Rosen, 2000; Wade, 1996, 1998; Wambach, H., 1981). To separate out consciousness from the human experience in our scientific pursuit to understand human experience and development, appears a "fatal flaw of the Newtonian scientific approach."

My present cosmology has evolved to view the primary journey as consciousness as *the* organizing principle of our human experience and journey. I believe our consciousness coming into this life has a unique shape with specific purposes for our life. Those may include grappling with certain limiting or destructive beliefs we bring with us to heal and resolve. They certainly are to grow, learn, enjoy, create, give, love, remember, and live more fully the Divine consciousness that we are.

I believe there is purpose and meaning in who we choose for our parents, the timing of our birth, and in our early prenatal and birth experiences because all these contribute immensely to the core beliefs and perceptions that begin to give focus to our exploration. From the very beginning at conception (and even before), we are learning about physical life through our experiences in the womb, resonating and merging with our parent's living of life and their conscious and unconscious beliefs. When we look at the states of consciousness and brain wave patterns of prenates and babies during the first eighteen months, it appears that we are "wired" as consciousness coming in to merge with the experiences of our parents and significant others. We enter an intense learning period about being human, about our own image and about the world; we form our personal perceptions and beliefs.

It would seem to be a beautiful plan to orient to our life in the physical world, merging our consciousness with mother and father's universes of biology and consciousness. We set the *filtering devices* that will determine what we consciously attend to and perceive. Out of the infinite possible experiences in human life, we begin to draw the core design of our life focus.

Unfortunately, all too often we forget that we are primarily consciousness. We have lost touch with life filled with soul and spirit and that conception is first and foremost a sacred initiation into life here. Sadly, we have narrowed our view of who babies are, based only on biology. In doing so, we have already abandoned their more real identity as consciousness capable of complex understanding and presence, as described by Chamberlain (1988, 1998, 1990) and Wade (1996, 1998). Our personal orientation and welcoming style has often become a school in separation, loneliness, toxicity, violence and fear, dimming the aliveness we knew outside the physical body (Emerson, 1996).

These early imprints and ensuing beliefs of human life can become our greatest constrictors—wardens of an inner personal prison—or they can be our greatest liberators. When we begin with belief that we are primarily consciousness, and that our physical self cannot be separated from, nor exist without, a connection to our consciousness, a whole world of new perceptions of what babies are showing us can unfold. As we begin perceiving the underlying beliefs that babies are portraying, we can begin working directly with those beliefs creating new possibilities of freedom, growth and health.

How Babies Portray Their Beliefs

Vignettes are useful in that babies are the best teachers to demonstrate the power of beliefs already imprinted. We also can learn from them as we watch those moments of new possibilities, when they move from constricted beliefs into beliefs that allow more freedom and growth. These vignettes come from the BEBA video archives. BEBA is a non-profit research clinic that I co-founded with Dr. Ray Castellino in 1994 to provide prenatal and birth therapy for babies and their families and to document the work for educational and research purposes. In the vignettes described, Ray and I are the therapists with BEBA families.

In therapeutic work with babies, babies show us how beliefs are more than thoughts. Beliefs permeate, influence, and are part of the very core of being at all levels: they appear as ways of *being* in the world, revealed in states of being, embedded and expressed in body structures, postures, physiological processes, and movement on both micro and macro levels. They also appear in states of consciousness, focuses of attention, emotional tones, and intentional actions. There is an *is-ness* to the experience, already a part of the fabric of being from which they live.

Remarkably, prenates and babies demonstrate to us that they do understand complex communication and respond meaningfully (Chamberlain, 1998). They taught me continually to stretch my "realm of possibilities" to include a knowing that this level of communication with babies was possible. I now recognize that it is possible because we are communicating at the level of consciousness.

How do babies communicate? They communicate through eye contact, facial expression, changes in where they place their attention and states of consciousness, body movements and gestures, physiological changes, breath and heart rates, vocalizations, crying and talking, through more primary changes in structure and rhythms and through energetic and telepathic means—i.e., a lot like adults do!

Principles of Repatterning

In the following vignettes, several repatterning principles are incorporated. Although this paper is not intended to be a thorough articulation of possible therapeutic interventions with babies, there are certain principles that are important to articulate here and that are therapeutic when being with babies in any intervention.

When an earlier experience has involved stress, trauma, or shock, the baby person has experienced some varying degree of disorientation, overwhelm and inability to cope in the situation (Castellino, 2000; Emerson, 1999; Levine, 1997). Events and sequencing were compressed and occurred very quickly or intensely. Each of the repatterning principles is designed to help babies repattern those earlier experiences by

190

supporting them to orient and to integrate present experience.

The first principle is to find the right pace for the baby. Usually this means we slow the pace as we sense the pace the baby needs in order to stay present and oriented, as well as connected to the slower more growth-oriented inner rhythms. This is an integral part of establishing a therapeutic environment in which the baby's autonomic nervous system can respond with settling and integration after activation has occurred (Castellino, 2000; Sills, 2001).

A second principle is to view the baby as the primary focus of and active participant in our interactions (if they want to be). We follow the baby's cues and respond to them. Often prenates and babies are "in reaction" to others and their environment or held on the sidelines of the adult conversation as they are "talked about." In contrast, we want to support their participation, their lead, and their communication.

A third principle is to attend to the baby's communication (verbal, gestural, somatic, and energetic) and attempt to recognize, acknowledge, and reflect for them the apparent experience, perceptions or beliefs, they appear to be expressing.

A fourth principle is to assist the baby to orient with aspects of their experience by pointing out and differentiating, such as, between then and now, or between their own experience and that of their parents. We may illuminate and voice what belief they are portraying, what they may believe is true in the moment, even though it is based on past experience, rather than the 'actual circumstances' in the present moment.

The fifth principle deals with our intentions and attitudes. We are attempting to bring awareness and support to provide the baby an opportunity of healing. This is different from *treating* a baby or conducting some test or procedure on the baby.

Sixth is to hold the vision of them as primary consciousness and that they are communicating with us on many levels and to respect their innate wisdom.

Seventh (and perhaps most fundamental) is that we bring our caring compassion for them. I believe love *is* the greatest healer.

These principles are incredibly powerful and are recommended as therapeutic guidelines in interacting with prenates and babies in everyday life (See McCarty 1996, 1997).

Vignettes

Anna

Anna was born at 42 weeks gestation after over 20 hours of active labor, induction with pitocin, and 4 1/2 hours of pushing. Her birth was finally assisted by vacuum extraction. When she was born, she was found to have aspirated old meconium and was taken to the NICU for assessment and intervention. After two hours, the mother was able to be with her in the NICU. Anna spent five days in NICU. She did well, but needed oxygen support, was given antibiotics and kept sedated. For purposes of clarity, I am distilling Anna's story to highlight our particular focus. Within the sessions though, we hold more of the complexity of the baby's prenatal and perinatal history.

We first met Anna when she was 3 1/2 months old. She initially looked very wary and frightened as her parents carried her into the therapy room. Ray spent several minutes slowly approaching her as we talked to parents. When he came close enough, he gently offered her his hand, after asking permission to do so from the parents. Anna showed several defensive reactions and signs of disorientation. Although she maintained eye contact, her eyes widens in a seemingly shocked expression: her body wobbled, she leaned back, pushed her legs out straight ahead of her, made increasing vocalizations that matched her other behaviors showing increased unease and wariness. Her system was activated in a fight-flight response. We paused, and I said, "Oh, moving back now." She made eye contact with me and her system quieted. Ray moved a bit and she looked away (another coping strategy). I said, "Oh, looking away." She settled again. We were being sensitive to her cues and acknowledging her responses. We were attempting to be quiet with our movements and attention. As we did this, her system settled and she could be more present.

At another point in the session when she was apparently reaching overwhelm, her strategy appeared to be to dissociate. She turned her attention to gaze into a design on her mother's skirt. She maintained her attention there. I quietly touch the skirt and said, "Oh, I see you looking there at mom's skirt." She made eye contact with me. I said, "Looking at me now." Her eyes went back to the fabric. The dance was to gently meet her where she was without expectations and to allow her to feel 'safe' in her coping strategies.

Anna's behaviors and responses in the first session taught us a great deal about the beliefs and expectations that were already embedded in her perceptions from her previous experiences of multiple interventions at birth and in the NICU. Her behaviors were meaningfully expressing fear and wariness. In our repatterning, we slowed the pace, acknowledged her responses, respected her boundaries, and acknowledged and supported her coping strategies. We supported her choices and boundaries. We continued to do this type of relating during the session. This was undoubtedly significantly different from her earlier experiences of medical intervention. During the following session, there was a marked change. She was already making much more contact with us, able to settle more and have fewer fearful reactions.

Makala

One of Makala's unique qualities is that she is quite a talker. Even at the young age of 3 1/2 months when we first began working with her, she was quite verbally expressive.

One of the patterns her parents had noticed was that Makala would find herself stuck, like in a couch, or she would be in the middle of the room on the floor and act as if she was stuck and couldn't move. She would become increasing upset, agitated, and mad. When we heard her birth history, the meaning of her pattern began to emerge. She and her mom had 36 hours of active first stage labor. During that time, Makala would have been feeling the pressure of contractions, but no matter what she did, there was nowhere to go because the cervix had not completely opened.

In this first session, she appeared to have recreated this as Ray was holding her. She was lodged in the corner of the couch with nowhere to go. The sequence described below begins at this point in the session. Mom was kneeling beside her holding her hand and being very present, watching her and listening to her. I was supporting her feet and Dad was also close by. In the sequence described below, focus on the mutuality in our communication and the meaningfulness of Makala's responses to us. We utilized several repatterning principles. We were recognizing, acknowledging, being with her, listening to her, reflecting her verbally and somatically. She was having wonderful contact with all of us. She was finally having her 'side of the experience' heard. It is likely that this was very different from her original birth experience.

Makala had been just "hanging out" with us for several minutes in this corner spot. She slowly got more activated, more arm movements and vocalizations. At one point Ray said, "We're actually re-simulating that time when you were stuck in there for a long time." I follow with, "And this time she is talking about what it is like and Mom and Dad are listening." Ray adds, "And you can see Mom."

Mom is looking right at her nodding her head. Makala continued to vocalize more emphatically and at one moment she appeared to say, "I can't get out of here."

Ray responded with, "It's a long time stuck in there." Makala vocalized and expressed more. She appeared to be working really hard to say the words to have us get it. Ray said, "I get it. Okay. I am going to say it out loud, "It was an awfully awkward tight spot. "

Makala responded with direct eye contact with Ray and said, "Yehhh." Ray said, "Yeh, awkward and tight," as he gently reflected that prior relationship with the pelvis with his hands touching her head and side of face. Ray continued, "Yeh, that's how it feels."

Makala said. "Yehhh." Ray responded with, "Yeh, awkward and tight," and again, Makala was really efforting to get words out and we heard what sounds like a somewhat 'gargled' sentence: "Yeh, I can't get out of here."

I almost immediately responded with "And you couldn't figure out how to get through there." With that, Makala immediately responded with a rather dramatic movement pressing her head into the tight spot. She began really moving her legs and pelvis up and down, but she didn't move forward.

I said, "And you were really trying to get through there." Ray added, "You were really stuck there." She looked directly at Ray and makes pushing sounds.

The interaction continued from here. This brief vignette portrays the level of communication and the beauty and integrity of mutual communication. She was telling us her story and we all were listening, reflecting, empathizing and repatterning as we journeyed together. (This sequence of communication can be clearly heard on the audio recording of the presentation this paper is based upon. See McCarty, 2001).

During that week, she continued to apparently express this pattern. During the next session, Mom reported she has repeated this 'stuck place-no-where-to-go' behavior with agitation and frustration at home. During a second session, Makala continued this pattern. Now even though there wasn't a womb, there wasn't pressure, there wasn't anything to stop her, she continued to create this position, again and again moving her legs, getting frustrated and mad, but not moving.

At one point during the session, Mom was on the floor with her legs apart. Makala was on the floor on her back with her feet against mom's thighs and she was again acting very frustrated and mad. At that moment, I said, *"You know, you could move your mad feelings into your feet."* Instantly, she pushed her feet into mom and propelled herself forward. All three of us were surprised. Mom opened her mouth in amazement and scooped her up to hug her. This was the moment of new possibilities and a new belief was born.

What unfolded after this was her expressing "I can do this!" She started mobilizing herself and moving around the room and started having fun in her body as she discovered she *could* move after all! One of the things we know is that in trauma we can become immobilized, feeling helpless. Makala had shifted to having joy and fun experimenting in her body with finding her energy, finding her fire. She has a lot of fire and now she could use it in an empowered way.

Lisa

Lisa teaches us another aspect of the origins of beliefs. We had been working with Lisa and her parents for sometime and we noticed that when she started to stand up, she had quite a peculiar way of standing up with her legs very far apart and her hips very unstable. It was quite distinct. We assumed it had a meaning and purpose, yet saw no physical reason for it. Where did this pattern come from? We asked her mom, " What was happening to *you* when you were ten months old?"

Mom related that she was in a body cast and a Stryker frame. Her hips were not fully developed when she was born and she wore a body cast for the first year of her life. It had a bar across to keep her legs stabilized quite far apart. In the frame, she was pulled upright at times and propped up.

We saw a relationship between mom's experience of first standing and her daughter's. This is an example of a belief that came out of the parent's experience during the developmental period that the baby was now in. When there is unresolved, charged material in the parent's psyche and soma, the baby may portray these held beliefs and patterns. The baby resonates with the belief and can carry and incorporate it into his or her experience. Lisa was apparently incorporating part of Mom's patterning even though she herself was not in a body cast.

Lisa's mom had not consciously worked with what she may have felt or needed during those months she had spent in the cast. In a later session with us, Mom brought in pictures of herself as an infant with the cast on. One poignant moment was when mom was describing the bar across and the position in which the cast held her, Lisa was on her back portraying the precise position. We suggested to Lisa that this was the way mom had to be because of her hips and the cast, differentiating between her mom's experience and her own.

In a following session, Mom chose to go inside and work with her own infant and be the receptive, supportive person there for her younger self. I was basically sitting with her and energetically supporting her as she went into her own inward healing journey. Dad was holding Lisa and Ray was supporting and tracking her energetically.

There was a synchronized dance between mother and daughter. As mom went in, Lisa went in. A short time later, the energy in the room shifted as Mom emerged. Mom reported that she had had a new energy that opened and moved through her body, especially her pelvis and legs. She remarked that she felt a significant shift in the energy, a healing shift with her young one feeling heard and assisted. As Mom came out of her inner experience, Lisa emerged from hers. As mom was describing her experience, Lisa stood up and moved to mom. Lisa stood next to her mom and clapped her hands smiling. We joined in and then noticed that Lisa was standing with her feet under her hips. The old pattern released and the new one had begun.

When we recognize, acknowledge, differentiate, and support the parent to heal their potentially unresolved material, the baby is freed to resonate with more life enhancing beliefs.

Sunny

Sunny was a little boy that we began to work with when he was six weeks old. At that point, he had never successfully breastfed. The only way that he would take his mother's milk is with a syringe next to the mom's hand dropped into his mouth. Everyone was exhausted. Sunny appeared very weary and was not gaining quite enough weight.

His history revealed that in the first 75 seconds of his life, he had a multitude of interventions. As his head was born, the physician saw that Sunny had a cord around his neck and brought the cord around. His body came out very quickly. He had a considerable amount of meconium on him. The doctor immediately, in a brisk, very no-nonsense way, suctioned him with a bulb syringe. He then quickly cut his cord and handed him to the pediatric staff. They took him to the pediatric bed and opened his airways up by extending his head back to visualize and suction him more deeply for the meconium. His Apgar scores were good, but he was taken to NICU for 'routine' procedures. His dad stayed with him. He was reunited with his mom over an hour later. *He never successfully breastfed.*

Those first moments, minutes, and hours after birth are incredible precious and vital for bonding, self-attachment, the establishment of

197

relationship, and successful breastfeeding (Klaus, Kennell, Klaus, 1995; Righard & Alade, 1990). In facilitating therapy with babies, I have come to appreciate much more deeply the power of those first moments in terms of imprinting beliefs and life patterns.

During the first BEBA session when Sunny was brought to the breast, he had a very distinct movement and activation pattern. When he started to put his mouth around the nipple, his head jerked back four times in a brisk decisive pattern. He then became increasing agitated, upset and escalated to where mom stopped attempting to nurse him.

During the second BEBA session, we explored Sunny's birth story in what I have come to call the "birth review." An important part of therapy with babies is when the parents begin to tell the story of the baby's birth. We take a great deal of care to include the baby and to do the review very slowly, carefully tracking the baby's response. We pause when the baby responds or activates, to acknowledge, reflect, empathize, allow the baby to energetically discharge any shock, help their potency build, and to allow space for their system to settle (Castellino, 2000, Emerson, 1999, Sills, 2001). When enough care is taken to build a supportive environment, the birth review can be a powerful therapeutic process.

Sunny was very present and quiet with his eyes closed lying on his stomach on Dad's lap. Mom was on the couch right next to them. Ray was positioned at Sunny's feet with his hand on Sunny's back making contact and tracking Sunny energetically. I was sitting close by tracking Sunny energetically also. As we ask the parents to talk about the birth, we encourage that slow, quiet sharing in a delicate way to match Sunny's quiet and receptive state. The process took most of an hour as we watched for Sunny's responses to the story being told. At times he responded with sighs, increased respiration, perturbation of his energetic system, mouthing and swallowing movements and sounds and also once, with a smile. When his parents spoke of his cord being cut so quickly, his system released some shock and he aroused with a startle, lifting his head.

As we progressed we became aware of his possible beliefs and confusions. In this vignette, a few key moments that illustrate his beliefs and our working with him around these are extrapolated from the birth review. This was a pivotal session in terms of understanding self-attachment, the imprinted disruptions in the process and the vital implications for breastfeeding and relationship problems that could ensue. For an in-depth piece on this that includes a transcription of much more of the session, read Castellino (1997).

Dad and Mom were describing when he was suctioned with a bulb syringe first and then again more deeply to remove the meconium from his airway. Dad said, "They were talking among themselves (the medical staff)… "It's below…' They were talking about the meconium." Sunny began to breathe faster as his dad spoke.

A few moments later Ray said quite slowly, "Okay. This is really important, Sunny. The reason why they did that was because they believed that you swallowed or breathed some meconium and they wanted to make sure that was not in your airway and they did it in a no-nonsense way." Sunny made throat sounds and his breathing sped up. Ray said, "Yeh, I know it felt like that…It was hard." Mom quietly adds, "And they didn't acknowledge your feelings either or treat you like a person." I add, "I'm sorry." Sunny swallows strongly. Ray responds, "That's right and you can swallow now."

A few moments later, I said, "And you can tell Sunny, that you are with Mom and Dad now. We are going real slow and you are included now…that's what sensations around your mouth and throat meant back then. They were hard sensations." Sunny swallowed and made mouthing motions.

Ray responded, *"You can suck now.* Sensations around your mouth can start to feel really different now as you start to heal. It can include good feelings, secure, connected slow feelings. It can feel and mean different things. It can feel really good to have mommy's milk; *your* milk. Going into your mouth and down your throat."

I said, "Momma's milk is really nourishing and good. Mom's milk is safe to go down. The meconium wasn't. That's why they needed to get it out of your mouth. I think there is some confusion about that. *Momma's milk is healthy, nourishing and good to go down. It's okay.* No one has to get that out. It is different now. It is different. A different fluid in your mouth…"

A few minutes later Sunny slowly opened his eyes and then began to root on his father's chest. His mom picked him up and brought him to the breast. Again, we were going very slowly and appreciating the delicacy of the moment. As he started to put his mouth around the nipple, his head bobbed back again, but not as strongly as in the first session. He began to get upset and activated. He was both reaching out to his mom with his hand and pulling away from her breast at the same time. His cry and expression voiced his angst.

I respond with, "Sunny you are here with Mom and not in the hospital. This is about feeding from mom's breast. And it can bring up some memories. I know you are remembering back then. There are a lot of mixed feelings about coming to the breast. It is different now. And when you are ready, you can find that out. When you are ready, you can find out that Mama's breast is different than back then. I know it is scary. It's scary. I know you don't know until you try."

Mom finally brought him up to be on her chest. He was reaching out with his hand as intensity of his angst increased and continued. After a few minutes of reflecting and empathizing, I made a more overt intervention. I matched his intensity and said, "I'm going to make a statement for him: I want to nurse so much, but it brings up so many feelings. It is so hard. It is so hard. I want to and it is so hard. It is scary." Sunny, I can see it brings up that scary place … and you don't know. It's scary to try again and to see if it really is different." Sunny immediately quieted and settled, raising his head and said "Yeh," as he rested his head on mom's chest.

The following week the parents reported two days after the session Sunny nursed for fifteen minutes for the first time. The next day he had been inconsolable and the following day had been "his best day yet," being more content, smiling, happier. Since then he nursed successfully.

At some later date, we watched Sunny's birth on video. It was stunning. As we watched the sequence of interventions, it was clear where Sunny's distinct head jerking motion had begun. The movement matched the energy, rhythm, and intensity with which the doctor had suctioned him with the bulb syringe. This interaction had been the first sensations and encounter in the outer world and first sensations associated with his mouth and throat. It became clear that when he started to put the breast in his mouth, these beliefs, these perceptions and patterned responses would be activated. We put that together with the messages and beliefs he was receiving about what fluids mean going into his mouth: *"They are unsafe and must not be swallowed."* All these interventions happened just as he arrived. They became part of the fabric and meaning of the journey of coming into the world and coming to the breast.

If we look at his birth through the eyes of a traditional Newtonian paradigm, we would focus on the medical interventions done as protocol to prevent infection. Yet clearly, Sunny shows us a broader impact of early intervention that needs to be addressed. Although Sunny's first weeks were very difficult, a new story began to emerge now. Utilizing the repatterning principles and understanding the power of our beliefs— that Sunny's behavior was based on meaningful beliefs of the world and that we could communicate together at levels of complexity far beyond what traditional models would suggest—Sunny was able to move into a more nourishing and happy life based on more life enhancing beliefs.

These stories stand for many others not told. Once we have the conceptions and perceptions to understand the *language of beliefs*, we can hear the stories babies are telling and respond to them in more healing ways.

In Conclusion

This paper has focused on illuminating the power of beliefs and what babies are teaching us. Our earliest experiences lay the *belief blueprints* of our reality. Babies show us their beliefs all the time because *they live in the world of their beliefs*. Their beliefs come from a whole constellation of influences beginning with their own consciousness and what they bring in, intertwining then with the beliefs already embedded in their genetic material at conception from generations before them. Beliefs also come from their parents—the guardians of their earliest experiences—from their parents' conscious and unconscious realms, their present and past, as well as from environmental factors, other people, and energies around them. During conception, pregnancy and birth, these influences form a rich constellation, a synergy of impact, as they become embedded in the experiences that form our blueprint for life in the physical world.

Although these early *belief blueprints* can become entrenched and continue for a lifetime, when brought to awareness and worked with directly, they are quite changeable. This paper portrayed one way to work with babies' beliefs. The new field of energy psychology is opening up more ways to directly access and restructure constricting beliefs into more life enhancing ones. In working with beliefs, we are accessing the very foundation of organization of our reality. We are able to work directly to recalibrate and reorganize at a primary level affecting us on multiple levels—physical, energetic, emotional, mental, and spiritual.

We can help babies repattern beliefs of constriction, fear, violence and separation into beliefs of connection and growth; beliefs that will help them experience the joy of living in a friendly, healthy world.

In his book, *Reinventing Medicine: Beyond Mind-Body to a New Era of Healing,* Larry Dossey, M.D. calls for an evolution of medicine (1999). He articulates three eras of medicine. Era I Medicine focuses on physical medicine and is rooted in the Newtonian paradigm, thus a mechanical view of the human being. Surgery, procedures, drugs are the means of intervention. Era II Medicine includes mind-body and looks at the impact of consciousness within the person on their health and well-being. Dossey favors a shift in medicine into what he has described as Era III Medicine. This era stands on the premise that we are primarily consciousness in human form and calls for the inclusion of a broader spectrum of human experience and therapeutic interventions. Dossey has reported extensively on the use of interventions that incorporate transpersonal skills such as intuition, distant healing, practitioner intention, and spiritual connection (1982, 1989, 1993, 1999, 2001).

I believe it is vital for those of us in the healing arts working with prenates and babies to broaden our views of babies and the ways we can help them, based on the premise that we are primarily consciousness. Many in our field have carried this torch for years, and I acknowledge and am grateful to them. Jenny Wade (1996) led the way in developmental theory with her groundbreaking transpersonal model of development that incorporates prenatal and perinatal psychology research and perspectives.

I call on the many complementary fields dealing with infants and infant development and intervention to incorporate consciousness in their conceptualizations and research. The next step in my mind is to translate what this premise means in terms of learning to read babies' language of beliefs and to relate with them at a whole new depth that accesses not only more of who they are, but more of who *we are* as well.

During the prenatal and infancy period, babies are beautifully open to learning and connecting at a profound level. Many of us spend much of our lives seeking to touch that potential again through love, beauty, solitude, meditation and prayer in order to re-connect with the Divine. Often though, because of our wounded beginnings, the pathway to our soul has been etched in sorrow, tragedy, and loneliness. What pathways do we want babies to have?

In those months in the womb and infancy, babies have the potential to develop pathways of growth and loving connection. Those early experiences deeply interweave the perspectives of consciousness as they transition to physical life, experiences that intertwine the physical and non-physical realms of experience. The more we can hold this richer perspective for the baby, the more this synergy of Self in human form can become the *beliefs blueprint* for life. When we hold this, the sacred journey of consciousness can again take priority and we can create more pathways of exploration of human life filled with deeper connections to the Divine, to self, others, humanity, and to the earth herself.

As the Beatles sang, "And the world would be a better place for you, for me. You just wait and see!"

References

Benson, H. (1996). *Timeless healing: The power and biology of belief.* New York: Simon and Schuster.

Bell, M.A. & Fox, N.A. (1994). Brain development over the first year of life: Relations between electroencephalographic frequency and coherence and cognitive and affective behaviors. In G. Dawson & K.W. Fischer (Eds.), *Human behavior and the developing brain* (pp. 93-133). New Guilford Press.

Bohm, D. (1980). *Wholeness and the implicate order*. London: Routledge and Kegan Paul.

Carman, E.M. & Carman, N. J. (1999). *Cosmic cradle: Souls waiting in the wings for birth*. Fairfield, Iowa: Sunstar Publishing Ltd.

Castellino, R. with Takikawa, D. & Wood, S. (1997). *The caregivers' role in birth and newborn self- attachment needs*. Santa Barbara, CA: BEBA. (Available through Castellino Training Seminars 805 687-2897)

Castellino, R. (2000). The stress matrix: Implications for prenatal and birth therapy. *Journal of Prenatal and Perinatal Psychology and Health, 15* (4) 31-62.

Castellino, R. (2001). Paper presented at the 10th International Congress of The Association for Prenatal and Perinatal Psychology and Health, December 2001, San Francisco, CA.

Chamberlain, D. (1988). The mind of the newborn: Increasing evidence of competence. In P.G. Fedor-Freybergh & M.L.Vogel (Eds.). *Prenatal and perinatal psychology and medicine: Encounter with the unborn, a comprehensive survey of research and practice*. Park Ridge, NJ: Parthenon.

Chamberlain, D. (1990). The expanding boundaries of memory. *Pre- and Perinatal Psychology Journal, 4*(3), 171-189.

Chamberlain, D. (1998). *The mind of your newborn baby* (3rd ed.). Berkeley, CA: North Atlantic Books.

Chamberlain, D. (1998). Prenatal receptivity and intelligence. *Journal of Prenatal and Perinatal Psychology and Health, 12*(3-4), 95-117.

Dossey, L. (1982). *Space, time and medicine*. Boston: Shambala Publications.

Dossey, L. (1989). *Recovering the soul: A scientific and spiritual search*. New York: Bantam.

Dossey, L. (1993). *Healing words: The power of prayer and the practice of medicine*. San Francisco: HarperSanFrancisco.

Dossey, L. (1999). *Reinventing medicine: Beyond mind-body to a new era of healing*. New York: HarperSanFrancisco.

Dossey, L. (2001). *Healing beyond the body: Medicine and the infinite reach of the mind*. Boston: Shambala.

Emerson, W. (1989a). *The power of prenatal and perinatal experience in maximizing human potential throughout life*. Paper presented at the Prenatal and Perinatal Psychology Conference, Newport Beach, CA.(January).

Emerson, W. (1989b). Psychotherapy with infants and children. *Pre- and Perinatal Psychology Journal, 3*(3), 190-217.

Emerson, W. (1996). The vunerable prenate. *Pre- and Perinatal Psychology Journal, 10* (3), 125-142.

Emerson, W. (1999). (Audiotape). *Shock, a universal malady: Prenatal and perinatal origins of suffering.* (Available from: www.Emersonbirthrx.com).

Klaus, M. H., Kennell, J .H. & Klaus, P.H. (1995). *Bonding: Building the foundations of secure attachment and independence.* New York: Addison-Wesley Publishing Company.

Laibow, R. (1999). Medical applications of neurofeedback. In J. R. Evans & A. Abarbanel (Eds.), *Introduction to quantitative EEG and neurofeedback.* San Diego, CA: Academic Press.

Lipton, B. (1998). Nature, nurture, and the power of love. *Journal of Prenatal and Perinatal Psychology and Health, 13*(1), 3-10.

Lipton, B. (2001). *Nature, nurture and human development.* Paper presented at the 10th International Congress of The Association for Prenatal and Perinatal Psychology and Health, December 2001, San Francisco, CA.

Luminare-Rosen, C. (2000). *Parenting begins before conception: A guide to preparing body, mind, and spirit for you and your future child.* Vermont: Healing Arts Press.

McCarty, W. (1996). *Being with babies: What babies are teaching us, an introduction,1.* Goleta, CA: Wondrous Beginnings. (Available through www.wondrousbeginnings.com).

McCarty W. (1997). *Being with babies: What babies are teaching us: Supporting babies' innate wisdom, 2.* Goleta, CA: Wondrous Beginnings. (Available from www.wondrousbeginnings.com).

McCarty, W. (2001). (Audiotape) The power of beliefs: What babies are teaching us. Paper presented at the 10th International Congress of The Association for Prenatal and Perinatal Psychology and Health, December 2001, San Francisco, CA (Available from www.conferencerecording.com.)

Ornstein, R. & Sobel, D. (1987). *The healing brain: Breakthrough discoveries about how the brain keeps us healthy.* New York: Simon & Schuster.

Righard, L. & Alade, M. (1990). Effect of delivery room routines on success of first breast-feed. *Lancet*, 336, 1105-1107.

Robbins, J. (2000). *A symphony in the brain.* New York: Atlantic Monthly Press.

Rossi, E. L. (1993). *The psychobiology of mind-body healing: New concepts of therapeutic hypnosis.* New York: W.W. Norton.

Sills, F. (2001). *Craniosacral biodynamics. Volume one: The breath of life, biodynamics, and fundamental skills.* Berkeley, CA: North Atlantic Books.

Talbot, M. (1992). *The holographic universe.* New York: Harper Perennial.

Wade, J. (1996). *Changes of mind: A holonomic theory of the evolution of consciousness.* Albany, New York: State University of New York Press.

Wade, J. (1998). Physically transcendent Awareness: A comparison of the phenomenology of consciousness before birth and after death. *Journal of Near-Death Studies, 16*(4), 249-275.

Wambach, H. (1979). *Life before life.* New York: Bantam Books.

Wilbur, K. (2000). *Integral psychology: Consciousness, spirit, psychology and therapy.* Boston: Shambala.

Wolf, S. (1950). Effects of suggestion and conditioning on the action of chemical agents in human subjects: The pharmacology of placebos. *Journal of Clinical Investigation, 29*, 100-109.

Appendix
The Resonant Heart

The Resonant Heart" by Rollin McCraty, PhD, Raymond Trevor Bradley & Dana Tomasino, published in *Shift: At the Frontiers of Consciousness* No. 5 (Dec. 2004-Feb. 2005), is reprinted by permission of the authors (www.heartmath.org) and the Institute of Noetic Sciences (www.noetic.org). Copyright 2005, all rights reserved.

Heart Fields

Heart Field Interactions Within the Body

Many believe that conscious awareness originates in the brain alone. Recent scientific research suggests that consciousness actually emerges from the brain and body acting together. A growing body of evidence suggests that the heart plays a particularly significant role in this process.

Far more than a simple pump, as was once believed, scientists now recognize the heart to also be a highly complex system with its own functional "brain." Research in the new discipline of neurocardiology shows that the heart is a sensory organ and a sophisticated center for receiving and processing information. The nervous system within the heart (or "heart brain") enables it to learn, remember, and make functional decisions independent of the brain's cerebral cortex. Moreover, numerous experiments have demonstrated that the signals the heart continuously sends to the brain influence the function of higher brain centers involved in perception, cognition, and emotional processing.

In addition to the extensive neural communication network linking the heart with the brain and body, the heart also communicates information to the brain and throughout the body via electromagnetic field interactions. The heart generates the body's most powerful and most extensive rhythmic electromagnetic field. Compared to the electromagnetic field produced by the brain, the electrical component of the heart's field is about 60 times greater in amplitude, and permeates every cell in the body. The magnetic component is approximately 5000 times stronger than the brain's magnetic field and can be detected several feet away from the body with sensitive magnetometers.

The heart generates a continuous series of electromagnetic pulses in which the time interval between each beat varies in a dynamic and complex manner. The heart's ever-present rhythmic field has a powerful influence on processes throughout the body. We have demonstrated, for example, that brain rhythms naturally synchronize to the heart's rhythmic activity, and also that during sustained feelings of love or appreciation, the blood pressure and respiratory rhythms, among other oscillatory systems, entrain to the heart's rhythm.

We propose that the heart's field acts as a carrier wave for information that provides a global synchronizing signal for the entire body. Specifically, we suggest that as pulsing waves of energy radiate out from the heart, they interact with organs and other structures. The waves encode or record the features and dynamic activity of these structures in patterns of energy waveforms that are distributed throughout the body. In this way, the encoded information acts to *in-form* (literally, *give shape to*) the activity of all bodily functions—to coordinate and synchronize processes in the body as a whole. This perspective requires an *energetic* concept of information, in which *patterns* of organization are enfolded into waves of energy of system activity distributed throughout the system as a whole.

Basic research at the Institute of HeartMath shows that information pertaining to a person's emotional state is also communicated throughout the body via the heart's electromagnetic field. The rhythmic beating patterns of the heart change significantly as we experience different emotions. Negative emotions, such as anger or frustration, are associated with an erratic, disordered, *incoherent* pattern in the heart's rhythms. In contrast, positive emotions, such as love or appreciation, are associated with a smooth, ordered, *coherent* pattern in the heart's rhythmic activity. In turn, these changes in the heart's beating patterns create corresponding changes in the structure of the electromagnetic field radiated by the heart, measurable by a technique called spectral analysis.

More specifically, we have demonstrated that sustained positive emotions appear to give rise to a distinct mode of functioning, which we call *psychophysiological coherence*. During this mode, heart rhythms exhibit a sine wave-like pattern and the heart's electromagnetic field becomes correspondingly more organized.

* At the *physiological* level, this mode is characterized by increased efficiency and harmony in the activity and interactions of the body's systems.

* *Psychologically*, this mode is linked with a notable reduction in internal mental dialogue, reduced perceptions of stress, increased emotional balance, and enhanced mental clarity, intuitive discernment, and cognitive performance.

In sum, our research suggests that psychophysiological coherence is important in enhancing consciousness—both for the body's sensory awareness of the information required to execute and coordinate physiological function, and also to optimize emotional stability, mental function, and intentional action. Furthermore, as we see next, there is experimental evidence that psychophysiological coherence may increase our awareness of and sensitivity to others around us. The Institute of HeartMath has created practical technologies and tools that all people can use to increase coherence.

Heart Field Interactions Between Individuals

Most people think of social communication solely in terms of overt signals expressed through language, voice qualities, gestures, facial expressions, and body movements. However, there is now evidence that a subtle yet influential electromagnetic or "energetic" communication system operates just below our conscious awareness. Energetic interactions likely contribute to the "magnetic" attractions or repulsions that occur between individuals, and also affect social exchanges and relationships.

Moreover, it appears that the heart's field plays an important role in communicating physiological, psychological, and social information between individuals.

Experiments conducted at the Institute of HeartMath have found remarkable evidence that the heart's electromagnetic field can transmit information between people. We have been able to measure an exchange of heart energy between individuals up to 5 feet apart. We have also found that one person's brain waves can actually synchronize to another person's heart. Furthermore, when an individual is generating a coherent heart rhythm, synchronization between that person's brain waves and another person's heartbeat is more likely to occur. These findings have intriguing implications, suggesting that individuals in a psychophysiologically coherent state become more aware of the information encoded in the heart fields of those around them.

The results of these experiments have led us to infer that the nervous system acts as an "antenna," which is tuned to and responds to the electromagnetic fields produced by the hearts of other individuals. We believe this capacity for exchange of energetic information is an innate ability that heightens awareness and mediates important aspects of true empathy and sensitivity to others Furthermore, we have observed that this energetic communication ability can be intentionally enhanced, producing a much deeper level of nonverbal communication, understanding, and connection between people. There is also intriguing evidence that heart field interactions can occur between people and animals.

In short, energetic communication via the heart field facilitates development of an expanded consciousness in relation to our social world.

The Heart's Field and Intuition

There are also new data suggesting that the heart's field is directly involved in intuitive perception, through its coupling to an energetic information field outside the bounds of space and time. Using a rigorous experimental design, we found compelling evidence that both the heart and brain receive and respond to information about a future event *before the event actually happens.* Even more surprising was our finding that the heart appears to receive this "intuitive" information before the brain. This suggests that the heart's field may be linked to a more subtle energetic field that contains information on objects and events remote in space or ahead in time. Called by Karl Pribram and others the "spectral domain," this is a fundamental order of potential energy that enfolds space and time, and is thought to be the basis for our consciousness of "the whole." (See www.*heartmath.org* for further detail.)

Social Fields

In the same way that the heart generates energy in the body, we propose that the social collective is the activator and regulator of the energy in social systems.

A body of groundbreaking work shows how the field of socioemotional interaction between a mother and her infant is essential to brain development, the emergence of consciousness, and the formation of a healthy self-concept. *These interactions are organized along two relational dimensions—stimulation of the baby's emotions, and regulation of shared emotional energy. Together they form a socioemotional field through which enormous quantities of psychobiological and psychosocial information are exchanged.* Coherent organization of the mother-child relations that make up this field is critical. This occurs when interactions are charged, most importantly, with positive emotions (love, joy, happiness, excitement, appreciation, etc.), and are patterned as highly synchronized, reciprocal exchanges between these two individuals. These patterns are imprinted in the child's brain and thus influence psychosocial function throughout life. (See Allan Schore, *Affect Regulation and the Origin of the Self.*)

Moreover in a longitudinal study of 46 social groups, one of us (RTB) documented how information about the global organization of a group—the group's collective consciousness—appears to be transmitted to all members by an *energetic field* of socio-emotional connection. Data on the relationships between each pair of members was found to provide an accurate image of the social structure of the group as a whole. Coherent organization of the group's social structure is associated with a network of positively charged emotions (love, excitement, and optimism) connecting all members. This network of positive emotions appears to constitute a field of energetic connection into which information about the group's social structure is encoded and distributed throughout the group. Remarkably, an accurate picture of the group's overall social structure was obtained from information *only* about relationships between pairs of individuals. We believe the only way this is possible is if information about the organization of the whole group is distributed to all members of the group via an energetic field. Such correspondence *in information* between parts and the whole is consistent with the principle of holographic organization.

Synthesis and Implications

Some organizing features of the heart field, identified in numerous studies at HeartMath, may also be shared by those of our hypothesized social field. Each is a field of energy in which the waveforms of energy encode the features of objects and events as energy moves throughout the system. This creates a nonlocal order of energetic information in which each location in the field contains an enfolded image of the organization of the whole system at that moment. The organization and processing of information in these energy fields can best be understood in terms of quantum holographic principles.

Another commonality is the role of positive emotions, such as love and appreciation, in generating coherence both in the heart field and in social fields. When the movement of energy is intentionally regulated to form a coherent, harmonious order, information integrity and flow are optimized. This, in turn, produces stable, effective system function, which enhances health, psychosocial well-being, and intentional action in the individual or social group.

Heart coherence and social coherence may also act to mutually reinforce each other. As individuals within a group increase psychophysiological coherence, psychosocial attunement may be increased, thereby increasing the coherence of social relations. Similarly, the creation of a coherent social field by a group may help support the generation and maintenance of psychophysiological coherence in its individual members. An expanded, deepened awareness and consciousness results—of the body's internal physiological, emotional, and mental processes, and also of the deeper, latent orders enfolded into the energy fields that surround us. This is the basis of self-awareness, social sensitivity, creativity, intuition, spiritual insight, and understanding of ourselves and all that we are connected to. It is through the intentional generation of coherence in both heart and social fields that a critical shift to the next level of planetary consciousness can occur—one that brings us into harmony with the movement of the whole.

For more information on the Institute of HeartMath's research and publications, please visit www.heartmath.org.

Address for correspondence: Rollin McCraty, PhD, HeartMath Research Center, Institute of HeartMath, Boulder Creek, California, USA. Phone: (831) 338-8500, Fax: (831) 338-1182, Email: info@heartmath.org

Index

About the Author

Wendy Anne McCarty, PhD, RN

Diplomat, Comprehensive Energy Psychology

Dr. McCarty is a leader in the frontier to support human potential and optimal relationships at the beginning of life and to support our evolution as integrated spiritual human beings of all ages.

She is a keynote presenter, educator, researcher, author, and consultant/mentor integrating prenatal and perinatal psychology, energy psychology, consciousness studies, spirituality, and primary psychology with her intuitive perception to inform, inspire, and support healing and transformation of practices and life patterns.

She brings expertise from her 30 years of professional work with individuals and families as an obstetrical nurse, childbirth educator, marriage and family therapist, and prenatal and birth therapist, as well as her current consultation practice for families and professionals.

She is the founding chair and faculty of the Prenatal and Perinatal Psychology Program at Santa Barbara Graduate Institute; the co-founder of BEBA, a research clinic providing prenatal and birth oriented therapeutic support for babies and parents; and, the director of Natural Family Living~Right from the Start, an organizational community to support human potential from the beginning of life.

To contact Dr. McCarty to bring this material to your community, or for your own private consultation, email her at:

wmccarty@wondrousbeginnings.com

To sign up for her free newsletter, see her upcoming events, and to purchase *Welcoming Consciousness* and her other products, visit her website:

www.wondrousbeginnings.com

CPSIA information can be obtained at www.ICGtesting.com
Printed in the USA
LVOW042030131111

254720LV00001B/16/P